Oral Probiotics

Fighting Tooth Decay, Periodontal Disease
and Airway Infections
Using Nature's Friendly Bacteria

By Case Adams, Naturopath

Oral Probiotics: Fighting Tooth Decay, Periodontal Disease and Airway
        Infections Using Nature's Friendly Bacteria
Copyright © 2012, 2014 Case Adams
LOGICAL BOOKS
Wilmington, Delaware
http://www.logicalbooks.com
All rights reserved.
Printed in USA
Front cover images © Befehr/Zentilia
Back cover "Vitruvian Man" by Leonardo da Vinci, est. 1487
Original illustrations by Virginia Callow
Anatomical illustrations (2) from "Gray's Anatomy" 1918

Publishers Cataloging in Publication Data
Adams, Case
        Oral Probiotics: Fighting Tooth Decay, Periodontal Disease and
        Airway Infections Using Nature's Friendly Bacteria

1. Medicine. 2. Health.
        Bibliography and References; Index

Library of Congress Control Number: 2009943532

Paperback ISBN-13: 978-1-936251-01-8

Ebook ISBN-13: 978-1-936251-02-5

Other Books by the Author:

ARTHRITIS - THE BOTANICAL SOLUTION: Nature's Answer to Rheumatoid Arthritis, Osteoarthritis, Gout and Other Forms of Arthritis

ASTHMA SOLVED NATURALLY: The Surprising Underlying Causes and Hundreds of Natural Strategies to Beat Asthma

BREATHING TO HEAL: The Science of Healthy Respiration

ELECTROMAGNETIC HEALTH: Making Sense of the Research and Practical Solutions for Electromagnetic Fields (EMF) and Radio Frequencies (RF)

HEALTHY SUN: Healing with Sunshine and the Myths about Skin Cancer

HEARTBURN SOLVED: The Real Causes and How to Reverse Acid Reflux and GERD Naturally

NATURAL SLEEP SOLUTIONS FOR INSOMNIA: The Science of Sleep, Dreaming, and Nature's Sleep Remedies

NATURAL SOLUTIONS FOR FOOD ALLERGIES AND FOOD INTOLERANCES: Scientifically Proven Remedies for Food Sensitivities

PROBIOTICS: Protection Against Infection

PURE WATER: The Science of Water, Waves, Water Pollution, Water Treatment, Water Therapy and Water Ecology

THE ANCESTORS DIET: Living and Cultured Foods to Extend Life, Prevent Disease and Lose Weight

THE CONSCIOUS ANATOMY: Healing the Real You

THE LIVING CLEANSE: Detoxification and Cleansing Using Living Foods and Safe Natural Strategies

THE SCIENCE OF LEAKY GUT SYNDROME: Intestinal Permeability and Digestive Health

TOTAL HARMONIC: The Healing Power of Nature's Elements

Table of Contents

Introduction

Every mouth is full of bacteria, yeasts, fungi and viruses. How do they get in? Simply by eating and breathing, or by putting anything into our mouths. With every breath, we breathe in thousands of airborne microorganisms. With every bite from every fork and spoon, we bring in billions of microorganisms from our foods, plates, cooking utensils and anything they may have touched. With every touch of a door handle or a pen or letter, we transmit billions of bacteria onto our hands, which make their way into our mouths when we wipe our lips, pick our teeth or blow our noses.

How can we stop infectious microorganisms from getting any further? Is there any way to stop them? Can we get them out with tooth brushing? How about with mouthwashes? What about dental floss, or fluoride treatments? How about with chlorhexidine (a popular periodontal rinse)?

We know by now that once bacteria get further into our body they can become systemic or septic infections. This is when the immune system may launch an inflammatory attack against the invasion, causing a variety of disease symptoms. This is where allergies, liver damage, kidney disease, heart disease, arthritis and many other infections arise. This is when conventional medicine is applied, with its arsenal of pharmaceutical antibiotic, antifungal, and antiviral medications. This is when the big guns of modern medicine get tossed into the ring, with their collection of side effects, adverse reactions and complications. This is when the astronomical costs of doctors, hospitals, urgent care are billed. And this is when the long-term damage to our intestines, livers, joints, lungs and urinary tracts gets done.

The fight rages on. Today we see millions of people dawning facemasks, washing with antibacterial soaps, and sanitizing classrooms, hospitals and other public places. This effort is not sustainable, however. We must find another solution.

Oral probiotics can provide that other solution. As we will show here, oral probiotics can be used to prevent infections from entering the body's internal tissues. Oral probiotics can line the mucous membranes, preventing or reducing infections of bacteria, viruses and fungi. Oral probiotics can also provide viable preventive measures for tooth decay, gum disease and those other infections that can result from microorganism invasions.

It is time to enlist nature's own enemies of pathogenic bacteria: our friendly microorganisms. Why reinvent the wheel? Nature has already provided the mechanisms that keep pathogenic bacte-

1

ria controlled for the most part: In the same way that populations of creatures within a forest balance each other through predatory behavior, our probiotic microorganisms keep pathogenic bacteria controlled within the body. Our stronger and more durable probiotic species will balance the aggressive yet vulnerable pathogenic species from growing out of control.

The battle between probiotics and pathogenic microorganisms has ensued over millions of years within the human body and other animals. Over this time, probiotic bacteria have been winning. How do we know this? Because humans and other animals are still alive! They have yet to be decimated by pathogenic microorganisms, long before man invented antibiotics.

While nature's balance does not necessarily completely remove the risk of infection, it goes a long way towards lowering those risks. It also offers us the opportunity to utilize nature's methods in a positive way to help prevent infection.

Here we will show that oral probiotics can strengthen our defenses against infection in a number of ways. They can help us reduce costly dental work and gum disease. They can help guard us against infection when we are traveling and among new environments.

It is time we employ our evolutionarily stronger probiotic bacteria—who have won the wars and battles against pathogens for thousands of years—to strengthen our immune system and prevent disease. We must arm ourselves, and fight fire with fire.

While some of the research and information provided in this book is also discussed in the author's book, *"Probiotics – Protection Against Infection,"* there are significant differences. This book focuses upon the bacteria and probiotic colonies that reside within our oral cavity and airways. Some of the same bacteria and probiotics that inhabit these regions also will inhabit our intestines, but many are specific to the oral cavity and airways; and most gain access to the rest of the body via the oral cavity.

Furthermore, oral cavity and airway probiotic strategies are quite different from intestinal probiotic strategies, and oral cavity infections create significantly different risks in other parts of the body.

Microbes in Every Mouth

Every mouth contains billions if not trillions of microorganisms. This is because we are surrounded by microorganisms. Trillions upon trillions of bacteria, fungi, viruses, parasites, nanobacteria and extremophiles live within our clothes, cars, bathrooms, beds, floors, air, and all over our bodies. Everything we touch has millions of bacteria living on it. Microorganisms also live in and around just about every food, no matter how much we cook it or freeze it.

Our bodies are also densely populated with bacteria. There are ten times more bacteria in our bodies than there are cells.

More than 700 different species of bacteria are residing within our mouths. These include species from the genera *Gemella*, *Granulicatella*, *Streptococcus*, *Lactobacillus*, *Veillonella* and many others. We each maintain unique combinations of these bacteria and others. In other words, no two mouths are alike.

Research has shown that thirty to seventy of these 700 or so bacteria species will be dominant within the mouth. This means that certain bacteria rule the roost. They control the biochemical environment, and the populations of their competitors.

At the same time, all of these different species live amongst each other in a cooperative, yet antagonistic manner. In other words, in a healthy mouth, there is a balance of bacteria, and the dominant species are probiotic.

Conversely, in a diseased mouth, the balance trends towards destructive or pathogenic bacteria. Multiple pathogenic microorganisms can grow and prosper within the mouth, teeth and gums. These include *Streptococcus mutans, Streptococcus pyogenes, Porphyromonas gingivalis, Tannerella forsynthensis* and *Prevotella* sp.

Additional bacteria can grow within root canals. Root canals provide protected spaces for bacterial colonization. Bacteria infecting root canals can include a variety of steptococci, staphylococci, and even dangerous spirochetes such as *Borrelia burgdorferi* among many others. Just about any bacteria that can infect the body internally can hibernate inside root canals. Because root canals are enclosed and the tissues around them die, the immune system cannot reach these areas to remove bacteria that may leak inside. As a result, a growing number of diseases are now being associated with root canal-harbored bacteria.

As these bacteria populations grow, they not only can infect teeth and gums with gingivitis: They can also cause inflammation and infection in other parts of the body. Infected gums have been implicated in a variety of fatal disorders, including heart disease, lung disease, liver disease, kidney disease, septic arthritis and others. A recent report from the Jos University Teaching Hospital in Nigeria (Adoga *et al.* 2009) reported that, *"Most often the cause of cervical necrotizing fasciitis is of dental origin."* Necrotizing fasciitis is a lethal infection of multiple bacteria that rapidly destroy tissues around the body, causing death very quickly.

Everything we touch has a way of getting into our mouths. Either we stick a fork or a pencil into our mouth, or we stick our hands in there to pick our teeth. We will wipe our lips with our arms and then lick our lips. Frankly, the mouth is the major gateway from the external environment into our internal tissues and organs.

The Germ Theory

Even though microorganisms have lived around and within humans and their relatives for millions of years, the past century has awakened mass paranoia and hysteria regarding the threat of microorganisms. Today microorganisms are considered one of the most critical threats to public health. After seeing the results of pandemics and epidemics over the past centuries—causing millions of deaths, our society has become focused upon microorganism threats in a profound way. Today, antiseptic soaps, antibiotics, mouthwashes, latex gloves, facemasks and many other antimicrobial devices are selling like hotcakes.

Still we do not seem to be winning this war on germs. Despite our antimicrobial technologies, contagious microorganisms are becoming increasingly aggressive and prevalent.

Today we are connecting more diseases to microorganisms. Is this because we didn't notice them before, or are they getting stronger? Coincidentally, superbugs and antibiotic-resistant microbes are on the rise. Autoimmune pathologies like Crohn's disease, chronic fatigue syndrome and others are also on the rise.

The following table illustrates some of the disease pathologies now being linked to microorganisms:

Disease	Microorganisms Suspected
Stroke and cardiovascular diseases	*Helicobacter Pylori* *Treponema pallidum* (syphilis) *Staphylococcus aureus* *Enterococcus faecalis* *Streptococcus* spp. Herpes Simplex (I and II) *Pneumonococcal aerogenes* *Candida albicans* *Streptococcus mutans* *Escherichia coli* *Chlamydia pneumonia* *Porphyromonas gingivalis* *Tannerella forsynthensis* *Prevotella intermedia*
Gallstones	Eubacteria *Clostridium* spp.
Ulcers, ulcerative colitis and Crohn's disease	*Helicobacter pylori* *Clostridium* spp. *E. coli* *Mycobacterium pneumoniae*
Cancers	*Staphylococcus aureus* *Enterococcus faecalis* *Streptococcus* spp. *Pneumonococcal aerogenes* *Streptococcus mutans* *E. coli* Mammary tumor virus Papilloma virus (HPV) *H. pylori* Heptitis B
Diabetes	Coxackle B virus Cytomegalovirus *Salmonella osteomyelitis* misc. bacterial infections (see below)
Arthritis	*Bacteroides fragilis* *Borrelia burgdorferi* *Brucella melitensis* *Brucellae* spp. *Campylobacter jejuni* *Chlamydia trachomatis* *Clostridium difficile* *Corynebacterium striatum* *Cryptococcal pyarthrosis* *Gardnerella vaginalis*

	Kingella kingae
	Listeria monocytogenes
	Moraxella canis
	Mycobacterium lepromatosis
	Mycobacterium marinum
	Mycobacterium terrae
	Mycoplasma arthritidis
	Mycoplasma hominis
	Mycoplasma leachii sp.
	Neisseria gonorrhoeae
	Ochrobactrum anthropi
	Pasteurella multocida
	Pneumocystis jiroveci
	Porphyromonas gingivalis
	Prevotella bivia
	Prevotella intermedia
	Prevotella loescheii
	Pseudomonas aeruginosa
	Pyoderma gangrenosum
	Roseomonas gilardii
	Salmonella enteritidis
	Scedosporium prolificans
	Serratia fonticola
	Sphingomonas paucimobilis
	Staphylococcus aureus
	Staphylococcus lugdunensis
	Streptococcus agalactiae
	Streptococcus equisimilis
	Streptococcus pneumoniae
	Streptococcus pyogenes
	Streptococcus uberis
	Tannerella forsynthensis
	Treponema pallidum
	Vibrio vulnificus
	Yersinia enterocolitica
Alzheimer's disease	*Chlamydia pneumoniae*
	Borna virus
	H. pylori
	Spirochete bacteria
	Herpes simplex I
	Picornavirus

Our microorganism paranoia began in the 1860s with Louis Pasteur's insistence upon the *germ theory*—a proposal that all disease was caused by microorganisms. To prove his point, he infected various animals with bacteria and studied their demise against uninfected controls. Yes, he proved that bacteria are involved in the pathology of many diseases, assuming inoculation beyond the capacity of the immune and probiotic immune systems.

He missed a critical element of the equation, however. Our entire planet is covered with infectious microorganisms in numbers beyond calculation. Each human body also contains trillions of microorganisms. So if the outside and inside world is covered with bacteria, why are we not all sick and infected all the time? How could some of us be healthy with so many bacteria around? And how could humans have survived this massive infestation of bacteria for so many thousands of years?

Microbiologists Antoine Bechamp and Claude Bernard, peers of Pasteur, took issue with Pasteur's germ theory. They proposed that the critical component in disease is not the microorganism, but the field or environment within the body. Bechamp and Bernard proposed that those who become ill had weakened and compromised immune systems.

In other words, a healthy body with a strong immune system and healthy probiotic populations is significantly more likely to counter and defeat infective bacteria.

We can confirm the field theory quite simply: Pandemic and foodborne outbreaks result in the sickness and death of not everyone, but sometimes only a few people—when thousands, even hundreds of thousands, may actually come into contact with the infective agent.

In fact, many of our foods host *Escherichia coli, Salmonella* sp. along with many other microorganisms, and do not make people sick. Most people can enter a hospital full of infected people and remain healthy. A few unfortunate visitors, on the other hand, may become extremely sick. Why them, and why not everyone?

Unfortunately, Pasteur's germ theory prevailed, and the genie of antibiotics and so many other pharmaceutical panaceas has escaped over the last century. While many of these medicines have helped millions resolve infections (after their immune systems recovered), the over-prescription of antibiotics and other pharmaceuticals has also destroyed probiotic populations and created numerous superbugs more powerful than previous species. In other words, the germ theory solutions have not stopped infection rates overall. They have actually created legions of stronger and more resistant microorganisms.

The Dawning of the Probiotic Era

The societies of the industrial revolution largely ignored the discoveries that proved the field theory and disproved the germ theory. In the first decade of the twentieth century, microbiologist and Nobel laureate Ilya Ilyich Mechnikov linked the longevity of the Bulgarians and Balkans with the eating of cultured dairy. Mechnikov was an esteemed scientist known for his discoveries of phagocytic white blood cells and their role in the immune system as they phagotize (break apart) invading microorganisms. Ironically, Mechnikov was also a colleague of Louis Pasteur.

After several years of research, Mechnikov proposed that tiny microorganisms living in the fermented milks drank by the Bulgarians were somehow stimulating their immune systems. His work with these microorganisms eventually illustrated that infectious microorganisms can be managed and controlled by probiotic organisms within the body. Over the past century since his research, many other scientists have confirmed and expanded upon Mechnikov's concepts. These researchers have found many more species and strains of probiotics, all of which contribute to strengthening the immune system and reducing infection rates.

The Anti-Microbial Mouth

Bacteria have been getting into our mouths for millions of years. For most of humankind's existence, we slept on the ground, earthen floors or straw beds. We farmed in our bare feet or in sandals made of rope. We defecated in holes in the ground and ate with our fingers. We drank out of the streams with our hands, and used twigs to brush our teeth. All of the microorganisms among these items eventually landed in our mouths.

This is more so the case among animals. Nearly every animal lives intimately connected to microbe-rich soils, waters and habitats. Virtually everything goes into their mouths. They lick each other and even bathe each other with their tongues.

Yet today, despite our various mouthwashes, antibacterial soaps, antibiotics and disinfectants, infectious diseases are on the rise. Rates of tuberculosis, influenza, shingles, mononucleosis, cytomegalovirus, malaria, HIV, AIDS and herpes are increasing worldwide. Estimates have calculated that 80% of the U.S. population may be infected with Herpes simplex 1, while some 45 million are infected with the genital variety, HS2. More than half the world's population harbors the *Helicobacter pylori* bacteria. About

1.5 million Americans are infected with sexually transmitted diseases gonorrhea, syphilis or *Chlamydia*. About one third of the world's population is infected with the tuberculosis bacterium, and every year about 6 million people die from TB according to the CDC. Millions more are infected with water-borne diseases throughout the world.

How do all these microorganisms get into the body and infect us? Most get in through the mouth. Either we breathe them into our mouths or we touch a doorknob and put them in later. One way or another, most infective microorganisms enter our bodies through our mouths, or nasal cavities.

Yet when it comes to our mouth, we are brushing with antimicrobial toothpaste, rinsing with antimicrobial mouthwashes, washing our hands with antimicrobial soaps and otherwise doing whatever we can to keep the mouth and the rest of the body as sanitary as possible.

Yet still we get cavities, gum disease and periodontal infections. Still we are suffering pandemics and epidemics. Still we are dying by the millions from microorganism infections.

Today American children receive more than thirty vaccinations for practically every type of infection with a history of risk to children. Adult vaccines are also on the increase. Today's vaccine line-ups include polio, measles, mumps, rubella, chickenpox, rotavirus, tetanus, pertussis, meningitis, diphtheria, hepatitis A and B, influenza, and now the human papillomavirus vaccine.

Most agree that vaccinations have reduced the incidence levels of many debilitating and fatal infections. Today, however, there is a critical backlash from a growing segment of American families. Many parents have begun to oppose the number and frequency of these vaccinations. Parents and reduced-vaccination advocates point to the dramatic increase of autism over the past two decades—from one out of thousands to one out of hundreds of children. Conventional medicine largely disputes this theory.

While this debate continues, there is no argument that microbial diseases garner significant attention from both government authorities and parents. Microbes are considered enemy number one by the Centers for Disease Control and government anti-terrorism officials. This outbreak and pandemic concern has been stoked by the many news headlines and journal reports highlighting fears of heightened death rates and hospitalizations.

The use of antibiotics has soared over the past few decades. Today, over 3,000,000 pounds of pure antibiotics are taken by humans annually in the United States. This is complemented by the approximately 25,000,000 pounds of antibiotics given to animals each year.

Meanwhile, many of these antibiotics either are given in vain or are ineffectual. The Centers for Disease Control states that, *"Almost half of patients with upper respiratory tract infections in the U.S. still receive antibiotics from their doctor."* This is despite the fact that 90% of upper respiratory infections and children's ear infections are not treatable by antibiotics. The CDC estimates that more than 40% of about 50 million prescriptions for antibiotics each year in physicians' offices are neither effective nor appropriate.

Indeed, the growing use of antibiotics has also created a Pandora's box of stronger microorganisms now referred to as *superbugs.* As bacteria and fungi are repeatedly hit with the same antibiotic, they learn to adapt. They learn to counter and resist repeatedly utilized antimicrobial medications. As a result, many microbes are stronger and more resistant to our antimicrobials. Like all living beings, microbes tend to adjust to their surroundings. If they are attacked enough times with a certain challenge, they are likely to figure out how to avoid it and thrive despite it.

This phenomenon has created *multi-drug resistant organisms.* Some of the more dangerous MDROs include species of *Enterococcus, Staphylococcus, Salmonella, Campylobacter, Escherichia coli,* and others.

One of the more dangerous of these superbugs is methicillin-resistant *Staphylococcus aureus* (MRSA). MRSA rates are on the rise, and nearly every hospital—the crown jewels of our antibacterial kingdom—is infected with MRSA. In a 2007 survey of 1200 U.S. hospitals, 46 of every 1,000 hospital inpatients were found to be colonized or infected with MRSA, with 75% of those being infected. Among the general population, the incidence of MRSA has skyrocketed from 24 cases per 100,000 people in 2000 to 164 cases per 100,000 people in 2005 (Hota *et al.* 2007). This means that MRSA is infecting nearly seven times the number of people it did in 2000.

The virulence of *Staphylococcus aureus* was first realized in 1929 by Alexander Fleming, a microbiologist who cultured colonies of *Staphylococcus aureus* close to growing molds. He noticed that the penicillin molds would kill some bacteria and not others. Fleming soon realized that *Staphylococcus aureus* adapted very quickly to the penicillin. *Staphylococcus aureus* became resistant. Even to this day, *Staphylococcus aureus* bacteria are still among the most antibiotic-resistant microorganisms.

Staphylococcus aureus is also one of the most lethal bacteria known to man. It secretes three cell-killing toxins: alpha toxin, beta toxin and leukocidin. Together these poisons bind to and dissolve cell membranes, allowing cytoplasm and cell contents to leak out. This, of course, immediately kills the cell. The immune system also has difficulty attacking and removing *Staphylococcus aureus* because it secretes enzymes that neutralize the immune system's attack strategies. *Staphylococcus aureus* adapts very quickly, so the more we throw at it, the stronger it becomes.

Shocking as it may sound, at the same time, most of us—even the healthiest of us—harbor *Staphylococcus aureus.*

Infectious bacteria are not always suspected—or even detected—in many diseases. Increasingly, we are finding that many common diseases are caused or worsened by bacteria or fungal infections. We are also seeing an increase in many degenerative diseases connected to infection—including cardiovascular disease, arthritis, ulcer, irritable bowel syndrome, asthma, allergies and chronic fatigue syndrome that appear connected to both yeast and bacteria overgrowth. Overgrowths of yeasts like *Candida albicans* can contribute to or be a primary cause for a number of diseases. Research has found that in some cases, *Candida albicans* can grow conjunctively with *Staphylococcus aureus,* resulting in the accelerated growth of both. This cooperative behavior between pathogenic microorganisms is technically called a *co-infection* in medicine. Co-infections occur in a variety of disease pathologies. We see this among the fatalities from influenza. Deaths often occur in immunosuppressed patients with concurrent bacteria infections.

Another resistant infectious bacterium is *Clostridium difficile.* This bacterium will infect the intestines of people of any age. Among children, this is one of the world's biggest killers—causing acute, watery diarrhea. It is also a growing infection among adults. Every year *C. difficile* infects tens of thousands of people in the U.S. according to the Mayo Clinic. *C. difficile* are increasingly becoming resistant to antibiotics and clostridia incidence is growing.

Pharmaceutical companies have produced hundreds of antibiotic medications. The reason there are so many antibiotics now is the same reason many pathogens are becoming resistant to many of our antibiotics: They are *static* strategies in a *living* system. Living systems are adaptive. They *learn* to work around whatever is thrown at them. Meanwhile, each antibiotic we have developed deters microorganisms with the same strategy every time. Some will interfere with the microorganism's cell wall. Others will interfere with the RNA within the cell—at least until they adapt.

How Do Bacteria Become Resistant?

A microorganism can learn to adapt to practically any threat to its survival, as can every living organism. In order to protect itself and its colony, a microorganism will gradually learn how to evade the threat. Over many generations, these strategies are passed on and perfected by successive genetic expression.

To illustrate how bacteria become resistant, let's say that that a burglar broke into a house while the family was home. The man of the house grabs a baseball bat and clubs the burglar on the head, and the burglar runs off. A month later, the burglar breaks into the same house again. What do you think the burglar will be wearing this time? A helmet!

We should understand that bacteria—even pathogenic bacteria—are living organisms that simply want to survive. Therefore, when they see a mass threat such as an antibiotic, over several generations they will figure out how to work around that challenge to their survival. They do this through the development of subtle and successive variations to their genes and genetic expression.

We might wonder how bacteria spread their antibiotic resistance. The interesting thing is that bacteria don't only create a genetic variation: They also create a small suitcase-like package of genetic make-over matter called a *plasmid,* with which they can pass on their genetic variation to other bacteria.

The plasmid is often called a *replicon,* because it can be transferred to another bacterium, who will automatically assimilate it into its genetic information. This allows the new bacterium to perfectly replicate the strategies of the source bacterium. Once inside the new bacterium, the plasmid allows the bacterium to perform the workaround to the antibiotic, and be able to pass the plasmid on to yet another bacterium.

Our broad-spectrum antibiotics might be compared to the baseball bat in the analogy above. Once used, bacteria may adapt to that static (antibiotic) tool. Any number of different species can figure out a way around an antibiotic. Once learned, that trick is passed on to other species of bacteria, and soon the antibiotic will be useless against many different species. This ability to learn on an inter-species level provides one of the scariest features about microbial infections: Their ability to grow beyond our ability to control them.

This also means that antibiotic resistance is not the same in all geographical regions. Plasmid transfer requires direct contact between bacteria. This was illustrated in a 2007 study on antibiotic resistance among several pathogenic bacteria. Gram-positive bacteria isolates were collected from 76 medical centers among nine regions across the U.S. The results indicated that vancomycin resistance in *Enterococcus faecium* ranged from 45.5% in New England to 85.3% in the East South Central U.S. Methicillin-resistant *Staphylococcus aureus* (MRSA) varied from 27.4% in New England to 62.4% in East South Central. Penicillin-resistant *Streptococcus pneumoniae* ranged from 23.3% in the Pacific region to 54.5% in the East South Central region (Denys *et al.* 2007).

This also means that as bacteria continue to travel on animals, humans, trains, buses, and airplanes, they will continue to exchange their learned resistance to our antibiotics. This will inevitably lead to most of our antibiotics becoming useless.

Probiotics provide the solution to this conundrum. How so? Probiotics are also smart living organisms. They are also the sworn enemies to pathogenic species. In fact, probiotics and pathogenic bacteria have been battling it out for billions of years, and the probiotics have been winning! This is evidenced, of course, by the fact that the human race is still alive. This means that probiotics have figured out how to identify each new plasmid, and respond by developing their own strategies and their own plasmids to combat pathogenic bacteria.

In our burglary analogy, when the burglar comes back in his helmet, the man of the house simply pulls out a new weapon with which to meet the burglar. If he comes back again prepared for that weapon, the man devises a new one. This is what living organisms do as they protect their territories: They get creative. As pathogenic and probiotic bacteria battle it out, they are both creating new strategies to resist each other. As one develops a new strategy, the other will develop yet another one. They both throw their biologically developed antibiotics at each other, and they each respond in kind.

Research has confirmed that probiotics have the same sorts of tools at their disposal. Probiotics can also develop antibiotic resistance just as pathogenic bacteria like MRSA can. Researchers from Sweden's University of Agricultural Sciences (Rosander *et al.* 2008) found that not only could the *Lactobacillus reuteri* probiotic strain easily develop antibiotic resistance: *L. reuteri* also developed plasmids. In fact, in their study they observed *L. reuteri* carrying *two* plasmids that created and passed on antibiotic resistance to tetracycline and lincosamide.

Foodborne Illness

It seems like once every few months panic grips us with a new outbreak of foodborne illness. The past year witnessed a number of big U.S. recalls and in recent years a variety of foods and beverages were pulled from shelves and restaurants after reports of sicknesses from foodborne bacteria.

Over the past two decades, we have seen a multitude of foodborne illnesses, the majority of which has occurred from meat.

Because meat outbreaks are so prevalent, non-meat outbreaks have become more sensationalized in the media. As a result, more products are recalled. The peanut butter contamination early in 2009 was the largest food recall in U.S. history, for example. After salmonella sickened a few hundred people, billions of dollars of foods—contaminated or not—with even trace amounts of peanut butter, were tossed out. During the summer of 2008, some salsa products were found to contain salmonella after they sickened a few dozen people. Two hundred hospitalizations and two deaths forced a huge tomato recall that dearly cost the tomato industry, though in the end Serrano peppers from Mexico were found to be responsible. In 2007, a listeria outbreak was blamed on milk products coming from a Massachusetts dairy. Two were said to have died from the contamination. A year later, 8,000 cartons of spinach were recalled after a few tested positive for *Salmonella,* even though no illnesses were reported. More sensational was the 2006 outbreak of *E. coli* poisoning blamed on spinach supplied by a California spinach grower. It was reported that three people might have died from the poisoning, and about 200 persons over two dozen states reported being sickened.

In 1999, *Salmonella* was also found in unpasteurized orange juice from Mexico. In one of the more sensational *E. coli* outbreaks, apple juice sickened sixty children with one death in the mid-

1990s. Other non-meat outbreaks of *E. coli* in the past few decades or so have included cookie dough, lettuce, and even drinking water. At the 1998 Washington County, New York Fair, over a thousand people were thought to have been sickened. Two people may have died from drinking the local water.

As mentioned, the majority of foodborne outbreaks are meat-related. These are no longer sensational news, however. Infectious outbreaks among meats or meat-containing products such as hamburger patties, pot pies, chicken, fish, beef, shellfish and many other meat products have infected people on a widespread basis for as far back as our media goes. *E. coli* 0157:H7 in beef alone sickens tens of thousands per year according to the CDC. Sixteen outbreaks in the past three years have been traced back to this pathogen in ground beef. During the summer of 2009 alone, 3,000 grocery stores in 41 states were subject to recalls of contaminated ground beef. *Salmonella* outbreaks have included chicken, scallions, and beef. Testing has also shown that 1 out of 20,000 commercial eggs are contaminated by *Salmonella enteritidis.*

Other bacteria also infect meat products. A *Listeria* outbreak infected thousands from chickens in 2002. Canned fish infected thousands people with botulism in 1992. *Staphylococcus aureus, Mycobacterium tuberculosis, Yersinia enterocolitica, Campylobacter jejuni, Cryptosporidia* and *Listeria monocytogenes* also infect meat products. Meat facilities can be laden with microorganisms, from rotting carcasses to infected food handlers. Certain viruses can also infect meat and fish products. *Calcivirus* or *Norwalk-like virus* infections have been documented, mostly from fish and oysters. Trichinosis, quite common in pork, can also seriously sicken. For this reason, food and health experts typically recommend that any animal products be cooked thoroughly before eating.

Ground beef is particularly vulnerable to contamination because, aside from the fact that a dead body naturally tends to decompose, most ground beef is made up of meat from different slaughterhouses in different locations, including outside the country. One study showed that commercially sold ground beef patties were a conglomeration of trimmings and scraps from slaughterhouses and processors from Nebraska, Texas, Uruguay, South Dakota and Wisconsin.

Few of these meat grinders are required to test for foodborne pathogens like *E. coli* and *Salmonella.* A study published in the *New York Times* found that many of the larger slaughterhouses even try to sell only to those processors that agree not to test their incoming meat for *E. coli,* for fear of setting off a large recall. Meanwhile, the USDA and FDA do little or no direct testing, relying instead upon the manufacturers to test their own products. Food safety expert and University of Minnesota professor Dr. Jeffrey Bender commented on this situation, saying that, *"Ground beef is not a completely safe product."* (Moss 2009)

These are but a few of the many recalls and outbreaks of food-borne bacteria over recent years in the U.S.

Does this mean we shouldn't buy and eat commercially prepared foods? Should we trust the inspection, pasteurization and sterilization processes supposedly supervised by the FDA and state health departments? In other words, can we trust our foods, and if so, which ones?

There are many reasons connected to infection occurrence, outside of the contamination and natural decomposition issue. One reason is that there is more mass distribution of food from one location to many locations throughout the U.S. This magnifies the potential for infection. Most food now travels well beyond outside of its current area of production, creating the need for increased storage.

Our ancestors were limited in their exposure simply because they were more in contact with their food. Their food was fresher. Now not only do manufacturers have to guarantee a food is safe after packaging, but they have to guarantee it through a lengthy journey through various distributors and warehouses, any one of which could contaminate or otherwise mishandle the product. This has forced manufacturers to come closer and closer to sterilizing our foods—and spoiling their nutrient levels—for fear of contamination.

Food contamination can come from many sources. The harvesting and plant environments, the cleanliness of workers, food washing techniques and water quality can all infect food. Bacteria can also reside within filling systems and packaging equipment, and within packaging materials. Even a sanitary facility can give rise to microorganisms, and these can get into the food during preparation. In the peanut butter recall, the walls and ceiling tiles of the peanut butter factory were found to be moldy. Surely, the mold did not appear suddenly on the ceilings. This means that people were eating contaminated peanut butter well before the recall.

As we compare the statistics between different countries and foodborne illness outbreaks in other countries, we find some interesting trends. Americans had 26,000 cases of foodborne illness for every 100,000 persons in the U.S. between 1996 and 1998. The UK had 3,400 cases per 100,000 people. France had 1,210 cases per 100,000 people. Why are Americans having more foodborne illnesses than the UK or France?

Let's analyze this further. In the U.S., 111 per 100,000 people were hospitalized for foodborne illness during this period. In France, 24 per 100,000 were hospitalized. In the U.S., 1.7 people died per 100,000 people from foodborne illness during that period. In France, .9 per 100,000 people died from foodborne illness.

The fact that there are more cases of foodborne illness in the U.S. per capita is overshadowed by the fact that there are so many more deaths and hospitalizations for foodborne illness in the U.S. per capita. It this caused by poor food manufacturing practices? Or perhaps it is something else.

Many species of bacteria can reside within any type of packaged food. *Clostrium botulinum* can grow in food or juice containers, especially cans, to produce a sometimes-deadly disease called botulism. *Campylobacter* species is one of the most common foodborne bacteria, usually prevalent among meat products. Still, this causes diarrhea, fever and cramping, but rarely death. The *E. coli* 0157:H7 bacteria can sometimes be lethal (verocytosis) in those with suppressed immune systems, but for most people it causes a little nausea and a few days of diarrhea. *Salmonella* is prevalent in the intestines of different wildlife, including birds, reptiles, deer and other animals (including humans). It too will mostly cause a little nausea and diarrhea in an otherwise healthy person.

While warm, moist environments are favored, bacteria can survive extreme environments. They can survive in the fridge, the freezer and even in low-oxygen vacuum containers. In colder temperatures, bacteria can incubate. A little warm moisture will revive billions of bacteria into colony formation. Many foodborne bacteria colonize via the release of spores, which can survive even the harshest conditions—including pasteurization. A single spore can quickly grow into an entire colony of bacteria.

Microorganism Mania

There are a number of different types of microorganisms within nature. Some are specific to certain environments, while others are more adaptive. Many of these organisms are only pathogenic should they grow out of control. Should their colonies expand beyond their normal boundaries, managed by the elements and other microorganisms, they can cause disease.

There is a variety of infective microorganisms. They range from the smallest fungi to elongated parasites, and everything in between. Here are the main classifications:

Microorganism Classifications

Fungi	Yeasts and molds; over 100,000 species; live in earth, air, water and damp, moist environments; can infect the body via food, water, air, and skin
Bacteria	Single-celled organisms; live in water, earth, air, on and inside other living organisms; can infect via food, water, air, and skin
Viruses	Non-living; genetic mutation triggers; exist in water, earth, air and skin; infect by altering cellular DNA, and spreading through ongoing cell division and mutation
Mycoplasmas	Ancient slow-moving bacteria; live on earth and water; infect mostly via food, water and touch
Parasites	Tiny organisms that infect and live within other living organisms. Includes worms, protozoa and amoeba
Thermophiles	Opportunistic bacteria that can live in very hot environments, such as deserts, boiling water or even in ovens
Psychophiles	Opportunistic bacteria that can live in the very cold, such as the arctic or in freezers
Nanobacteria	Extremely small bacteria that typically have a hard calcium shell. Thought to cause some diseases considered autoimmune.

Today we deal with a multitude of infections from all of these types of microorganisms. Growing infectious diseases from this list include tuberculosis, pneumonia, staphylococcus, streptococcus, *E. coli*, cholera, listeria, salmonella, shigella, dengue fever, influenza, yellow fever, cryptosporidiosis, hepatitis, rabies, Lyme disease and others. Many of these microorganisms are growing despite specific antibiotic and antiviral medications. Some are growing because of unsafe sex, unclean water or changes in land use. Many are growing because of new opportunities arising from our destruction of nature's balancing mechanisms.

How Many Bacteria Does it Take to Get Sick?

Most of us have a false sense of security in our antimicrobial strategies. We think that our antibiotics, antiseptic soaps and face-masks will keep us microbe-free. This is far from reality.

Let's look at pasteurization, for example. Louis Pasteur developed pasteurization in the 1860s to disprove the notion of spontaneous generation—a theory that some scientists of the day had put forth to explain how life arose from chemicals. Pasteurization is still the central antimicrobial strategy that commercial food manufacturers use to try to eliminate microorganisms from our foods and beverages. Is this strategy successful? Our outbreak record says otherwise.

Today pasteurization is used for practically every commercially packaged food that has significant water or moisture content. This includes nearly every shelf-stable canned food, sauce and mix in jars. Today even vegetables, nuts, fruit, pre-packaged dinners, entrees, and refrigerated juices are pasteurized.

Pasteurization is the attempt to remove microbes through either heat, chemical or electromagnetic means. There are five basic types of pasteurization: *Holder* or *steam* pasteurization, *high temperature* or *flash* pasteurization, *ultra high temperature* pasteurization, *irradiation* pasteurization, and *gas* pasteurization.

None of these actually will sterilize a food or beverage, however. Complete sterilization is extremely difficult even in laboratory conditions, and thus the term "sterilized" is seldom if ever legitimately used in food manufacturing. Depending upon the method, pasteurization will lower bacteria counts down by about 99%. This means, for example, if there were one trillion bacteria colony-forming units (CFU) in the food before pasteurization, there might still be ten billion CFU left after pasteurization. For UHT pasteurization, the removal rate can be higher; up to a 99.9% removal. This means for a one trillion CFU initial population, there would be one billion CFU left after this less-used and most-intense form of pasteurization.

How many colony-forming units does it take of an aggressive bacteria species to make an immunosuppressed person sick? One hundred? Ten thousand? A million? In the right conditions, any of these counts can expand into an aggressive, disease-causing colony of bacteria. A billion is certainly plenty: Assuming a suitable environment within which to grow.

The Oral Immune System

Friendly bacteria make up approximately 70% of our immune system and a healthy mouth is full of probiotics. The majority of our probiotics live in colon, although billions also live in the mouth and the small intestines. Other populations of probiotic bacteria and fungi can live within the nasal cavity, on the skin, in the throat, in the lungs, in the conjunctiva of the eyes, under the armpits, under the toenails, in the vagina, between the toes; and among the body's various other nooks and cavities.

The rest of the immune system is located throughout the body. We find immune cells such as T-cells, B-cells and immunoglobulins on the skin, in the blood, in the lungs, in the bones and in every organ system. We also find the immune system within trillions of probiotic bacteria scattered around the body. In fact, research has confirmed that over 70% of a healthy body's immune system is comprised of our probiotic bacteria.

Harmful microbes or toxins typically invade the body via the mouth or the nasal cavity. Other entry pathways include the skin, the genitals, the ears and the eyes. These entries, however, are less significant than the mouth. The oral and nasal cavities provide almost instant access to our internal organs and tissues.

Should pathogens gain access, our body's immune system has a number of intelligent abilities. The first is recognition. The immune system has the facility to recognize molecules that endanger the body's welfare. The immune system also maintains memory. The immune system can remember the identity of a toxin or pathogen by virtue of recognizing its antigens (byproducts or molecular structure). This is the rationale for vaccination. Vaccination exposes the body to a small amount of a particular pathogen so the immune system will develop the tools and the memory to recognize its antigens, enabling the body to respond appropriately the next time it is exposed to the same pathogen.

The immune system maintains specificity and diversity at the same time. These abilities allow the immune system to respond to literally millions, if not billions of different antigens presented by various microorganisms. Each particular antigen requires a completely different response, requiring the immune system to remember not only the antigen, but also the appropriate response.

The immune system's intelligent scanning and review processes gauge whether a particular molecule, cell or organism belongs in the body. This is determined through a multitude of complex biochemical identification systems. We might compare these systems to an iris scan, often used as a password entry system. Utilizing a database of information, the immune system checks molecular structures against this database. If the molecular structure isn't recognized, or matches a structure considered foreign, the immune system launches an inflammatory attack. This attack is referred to as an immune response.

This scanning and memory system is not entirely done by the various immune memory cells, however. Probiotics play a large role in scanning for abnormalities, and discovering invaders.

The body's memory and recognition system is extremely complex. Most medical literature tries to simplify it in order to allow us to wrap our minds around it. Here we also will only graze the surface, but we will introduce and review the element that has been largely overlooked amongst immune system literature: The role of the probiotics.

Let's review the immune system's main processes in general before we hone in on the role probiotics play:

The Non-specific Immune System

The non-specific immune system utilizes a network of barriers that prevent infective agents from getting into the body. These barrier structures include the facilities our eyes, mouths, noses and ears have to halt or shut out invaders or toxins before they can enter the body. These facilities include mucous, nose hairs, eyelashes, lips, teeth, tonsils, ear hair, pubic hair and even conscious tools such as our hands as we attempt to brush aside or block dust and other toxins. The non-specific facilities include the ability to close our mouths. They also include the ability to breath through our noses. Utilizing these facilities allows us to redirect or block the passage of dust, dander, and even microbial invasions before they can venture any further.

Our nasal cavities contain an intricate sequence of chambers with traps and narrow sections that provide an advanced filtration system. Each chamber is strategically placed, requiring our incoming air to travel through each chamber. This allows the filtering components of the nasal cavity to trap and remove any particles and microorganisms that may be contained within that air.

In addition, the surfaces (epithelium) inside the mouth and nasal cavity are covered with a thin liquid mucous membrane. This membrane maintains a unique biochemical mixture called mucopolysaccharides that can slow invaders as they attempt to penetrate the body and its tissues. Assuming a strong and vibrant immune system, this mucus lining will trap microorganisms and toxins into a snare of immune cells and immunoglobulins, along with, of course, colonies of probiotics.

The nasal cavity and parts of the oral cavity are also equipped with tiny hairs called cilia. Cilia help trap and evacuate invaders by moving rhythmically, sweeping back and forth, in order to move trapped pathogens outward with their undulations.

The digestive tract is equipped with another type of sophisticated non-specific defense technology. Should any foreigners get through the lips, teeth, tongue, hairs, mucous membranes and cilia to sneak down the esophagus, they then must contend with the digestive acidity of the stomach. The gastrin, peptic acid and hydrochloric acid within a healthy stomach maintain a pH of around two. This is typically enough acidity to kill or disrupt many microorganisms. However, a person can mistakenly weaken this protective acid by taking antacids or acid-blockers. In this case, the stomach's ability to neutralize pathogens will be handicapped. In addition, a number of microorganisms are accustomed to acidic environments, and still others can tuck away into clumps of food—especially food that has not been chewed well enough.

Humoral Immune Response

The second form of immune response involves a highly technical strategic analysis that first identifies the invader's weaknesses, followed by a precise and immediate offensive attack to exploit those weaknesses. This is often called humoral immunity. Here there are more than a billion different types of antibodies, macrophages and other immune cells that can be mobilized to execute specific attack plans. As an immune cell scans a particular invader, it may recognize a particular biomolecular or behavioral weakness within the toxin or pathogen. Upon recognizing this weakness, the immune system will devise a unique plan to exploit this weakness. It may launch a variety of possible attacks, using a combination of specialized B-cells (or B-lymphocytes) in conjunction with specialized antibodies.

Cruising through the mucous, blood and lymph systems, the antibodies and/or B-cells can quickly sense and size up viruses, toxins or bacteria. Often this will mean the antibody will lock onto or bind to the invader to extract critical genetic information. This process will often draw upon databases held within certain helper B-cells that memorize vulnerabilities. The specific vulnerability is often revealed by molecular structures of pathogenic cell membranes. Each pathogen will be identified by these unique structures or antigens. The B-cell then reproduces a specific antibody designed to record and communicate that information to other B-cells through biochemical signalling. This allows for a constant tracking of the location and development of pathogens, allowing B-cells to manage and constantly assess the response.

Cell-Mediated Immune Response

The third system used by the immune system is the cell-mediated immune response. This also incorporates a collection of smart white blood cells, called T-cells. T-cells and their surrogates wander the body scanning the body's own cells. They are seeking cells that have become infected or otherwise damaged by viruses, bacteria, fungi or toxic free radicals. Infected cells are typically identified by special marker molecules (antigens) that sit atop their cell membranes. These antigens have particular molecular arrangements that signal roving T-cells of the damage that has occurred within the cell. Once a damaged cell has been recognized, the cell-mediated immune system will launch an inflammatory response against the cell. This response will typically utilize a variety of cytotoxic (cell-killing) cells and helper T-cells. These types of immune cells will often directly kill the damaged cell by inserting toxic chemicals into it. Alternatively, the T-cell might send signals into the damaged cell, switching on the cell's own self-destruct mechanism.

The Probiotic Immune Response

The fourth and most powerful part of the immune system occurs among the body's probiotics. The human body can house more than 32 billion beneficial and harmful bacteria and fungi at any particular time. When beneficial bacteria are in the majority, they constitute up to 70-80% of the body's immune response.

This probiotic immune response occurs both in an isolated manner and in conjunction with the other systems of the immune system discussed above.

Probiotic colonies work with the body's internal immune system to organize strategies that prevent toxins and pathogenic microorganisms from harming the body. Once they identify an overgrowth, probiotics will communicate and cooperate with the immune system to organize cooperative strategies. They will also stimulate the body's immune cells, activating the cell-mediated response, the humoral response, and indirectly, the body's exterior barrier systems through mechanical stimulation (e.g., stimulating the production of histamine, causing sneezing). As we will see in the research, they stimulate T-cells, B-cells, macrophages and NK-cells with smart messages that promote specific immune responses. They also activate cytokines and phagocytic cells directly to coordinate their intelligent immune response.

Probiotics can also quickly identify harmful bacteria or fungal overgrowths and work directly to eradicate them. This process may not directly involve the rest of the immune system. Even still, the immune system will be notified of any probiotic offensives. The immune system will provide support for the process by breaking up and escorting killed pathogens and their endotoxins out of the body.

Probiotics produce chemical substances that destroy invading microorganisms. Probiotics make up our body's own antibiotic system. Because probiotics are extremely intelligent and want to survive, they have developed various strategies to defend their homeland (our body). It is a territorial issue. Invading bacteria threaten their homes and families. Probiotics also learn how to fight newer bacteria species and new bacteria strategies. While static pharmaceutical antibiotics are counteracted by smart superbugs, probiotics can alter their antibiotic strategies as needed. Our continued survival illustrates their intelligence in maintaining their hosts over time.

Probiotics produce antimicrobial biochemicals that manage, damage or kill pathogenic microorganisms. In some cases, they will simply overcrowd the invaders with biochemistry and populations to limit their growth. In other cases, they will secrete chemicals into the fluid environment to eradicate large populations. In still other cases, they will insert specific chemicals into the invaders, which can directly kill them or dissolve their cell membranes.

Probiotic mechanisms are quite complex and variegated to say the least.

Dr. Mechnikov hypothesized that the beneficial effects of lactobacilli arise from the lactic acid they excrete. Indeed, the lactic acid produced by *Lactobacillus* and *Bifidobacteria* species sets up the ultimate pH control in our mouths, upper respiratory tract and intestines to repel antagonistic organisms. Lactic acids are not alike, however. There are different lactic acid molecular structures, and combinations with other chemicals. For example, some probiotics produce an L(+) form of lactic acid and other probiotics may produce the D(-) from. Many probiotic strains also produce a molecular combination with hydrogen peroxide called lactoperoxidase.

Probiotics also produce acetic acids, formic acids lipopolysaccharides, peptidoglycans, superantigens, heat shock proteins and bacterial DNA—all in precise portions to nourish each other, inhibit challengers and/or benefit the host.

Precision and proportion is the key. For example, some bifidobacteria will secrete a 3:2 proportion of acetic acid to lactic acid in order to barricade certain pathogenic bacteria.

Probiotics also secrete a number of key nutrients crucial to their hosts. These include B vitamins such as pantothenic acid, pyridoxine, niacin, folic acid, cobalamin and biotin, and crucial antioxidants such as vitamin K.

Probiotics can also produce antibacterial molecules called bacteriocins. *Lactobacillus plantarum* produces lactolin. *Lactobacillus bulgaricus* secretes bulgarican. *Lactobacillus acidophilus* can produce aciophilin, acidolin, bacterlocin and lactocidin. These and other antibacterial substances equip probiotic species with territorial mechanisms to combat and reduce pathologies related to *Shigella, Coliform, Pseudomonas, Klebsiella, Staphylococcus, Clostridium, Escherichia* and other infective genera. Furthermore, antifungal biochemicals from the likes of *L. acidophilus, B. bifidum, E. faecium* and others also significantly reduce fungal outbreaks caused by *Candida albicans*.

These types of antimicrobial tools give probiotics the ability to counter the mighty *H. pylori* bacterium—known to be at the root of a majority of ulcers. *H. pylori* inhibition has been observed in studies on *L. acidophilus, L. rhamnosus, L. rhamnosus, Propionibacterium freudenreichii* and *Bifidobacterium breve.*

Furthermore, probiotics will specifically stimulate the body's own immune system to attack pathogens. For example, scientists from Finland's University of Turku (Pessi *et al.* 2000) gave nine atopic dermatitis children *Lactobacillus rhamnosus* GG for four weeks. They found that serum cytokine IL-10 levels specific to the infection increased following probiotic consumption.

Whatever the strategy, smart probiotic microorganisms work collectively and synergistically with the other three components of our immune system. Our probiotic system works within the non-specific immune system to help protect the body from invasions. Probiotics live within the oral cavity, the nasal cavity, the esophagus, around the gums, and in pockets of our pleural cavity (surrounding our lungs). They dwell within our stomach, within our intestines, within the vagina and around the rectum, and amongst other pockets of tissues. This means that for bacteria to invade the bloodstream, they must first get through legions of probiotic bacteria that populate those entry channels—assuming a healthy body of course.

Oral and Nasal Immunity

We find all four of the immune response systems active within the upper respiratory tract, which includes the oral cavity, the nasal cavity, the pharynx, and parts of the pleural cavity. This is because the mouth and nose provide one of the most accessible areas for microorganism and toxin entry.

Most of these systems require good probiotic colonies to be successful, however. This is because probiotics not only are part of the body's second line of defense: Their presence is essential for our immune response systems to work effectively.

The nasal cavity contains a labyrinth of various canals and chambers that allow any air we' breath to have plenty of contact with the mucous membranes and cilia of the nasal cavity. It was only until recently that researchers became aware that these various chambers housed more than mucous membranes and immune cells: They also hosted legions of probiotic colonies.

These probiotic colonies are saturated throughout the mucous membrane. Here they not only help identify invaders, but they launch their own attacks against invading bacteria, viruses and fungi. They will also translocate between different nasal cavities, the mouth, the pharynx and other regions of the respiratory system.

Olfactory bulbs are positioned mostly at the top of the sinus cavity on either side of the nasal septum. Olfactory bulbs lie at the epithelium mucosa surface, where nerve fibers connect to the bulbs. These nerve fibers sense the waveform and polarity of odorous molecules traveling in the air as they interface with the mucosa of the nasal cavity. These 'odor-packets' traveling within and around gas and air molecules stimulate the nerves in the olfactory bulbs.

Special olfactory nerve bulbs collectively called the *vomeronasal organ* (VNO)—also called *Jacobson's organ*—may be stimulated on a more subtle level by pheromones. Pheromones carry and exchange information through the environment between living organisms. Pheromones have been shown to stimulate sexual and reproductive responses among animals, plants and insects. There is some debate as to whether humans also exchange pheromones. While humans have anatomical VNOs—known for pheromone exchanging in animals—significant nerve conduction has yet to be confirmed physically. The assumption has been that without obvious VNO nerve pathways there would be little chance of information conduction to responsive endocrine or cognitive mechanisms.

Consideration might be given to the work of a well-respected rhinologist Dr. Maurice Cottle. Dr. Cottle, known for his contribution towards the development of the electrocardiogram, invented a diagnostic machine in the mid-twentieth century called the *rhinomanometer.* Dr. Cottle wrote two books on the subject of rhinomanometry, and was a professor and head of Otolaryngology at the Chicago Medical School. Dr. Cottle was able to diagnose a number of ailments in other parts of the body simply by measuring the swelling or shrinking of the tissues and the airflow through this region during breathing.

The delicate turbinate membranes are more than mucous membranes: They are erectile, with thousands of tiny receptors. They respond to stimulation just as do other erectile regions. The turbinate erectile receptors respond to and coordinate airflow with the rest of the body. Clinical evidence demonstrated that Dr. Cottle's machine could accurately diagnose coronary heart disease, for example.

In reviewing the connection between oral bacteria and cardiovascular disease, we find that the inflammatory response stimulated by pathogenic bacteria through the NK-kappa mechanism could also be at the root of the phenomena that Dr. Cottle was observing. An inflamed turbinate and sinus area would likely be the result of an imbalance of pathogenic and probiotic bacteria, causing not only cardiovascular inflammation as has been shown in modern research, but the swelling of nasal membranes like the turbinates. This swelling indicates an abnormality among microorganisms that inhabit the upper respiratory tract, likely mirroring further imbalances among the probiotic and pathobiotic microorganisms in the intestines and other regions of the body.

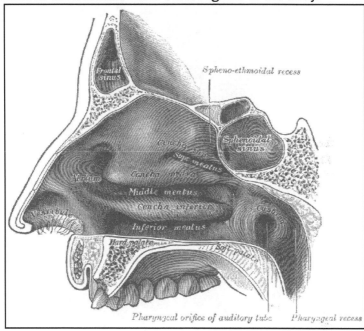

The Nasal Cavity

We can see some of these chambers from the above Gray's rendering. At the nasal entry, we see the atrium, then the middle and inferior meatus, separated by the concha inferior. Above these two chambers lie the septum meatus and then the sphenoidal sinus. These different passageways provide plenty of traps and filters to catch foreign particles and microorganisms. They also provide warm and moist nesting areas for our probiotics.

Once foreigners are trapped, these colonies of probiotics, along with our immunoglobulins and various immune cells, can corner them and break them apart—assuming a vibrant immune system and strong probiotic colonies.

Within the mouth, we also find various chambers and traps. The entire oral cavity is lined with mucous membranes that help trap microorganisms. Instead of cilia, however, the mouth has teeth, gums, and a big scaly tongue to trap and block particles and microorganisms. Once trapped, again, our probiotics and immune cells take control of foreigners.

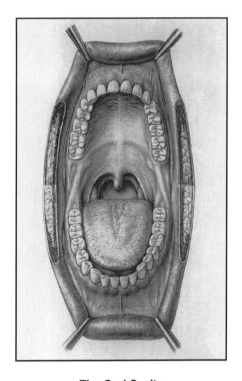

The Oral Cavity

Unlike the stable cavities of the nasal region, the oral cavity's trapping systems are also movable. A person can consciously move the lips, the tongue, and the cheeks to evade and trap particles and microorganisms. The tongue can also ferret out pockets of microorganisms from crevices around the gum line. This can be augmented with water, a toothbrush, floss and/or water irrigation.

The versatile tongue also has a surface that can trap microbes and particles. On the tongue's top surface are a variety of papillae and small bumps called taste buds. Together with a coating of saliva, this surface serves to not only channel food in and taste food: The tongue's surface also traps particles and microbes.

As we continue back into the oral cavity and into the pharynx, we find more mucous membranes, along with cilia. As we go deeper, we final the tonsils, which create a further trap or barrier for pathogens. As we will discuss later, there is reason to believe that the tonsils provide an incubation chamber of sorts for our resident probiotic strains.

Along with probiotic colonies, all of the oral, nasal and pharangeal mucosal membranes are coated with the humoral immune system. Here we find legions of immunoglobulins (mostly of the IgA type) and B-cells, which together scan and identify various types of microorganisms that are trying to get past our probiotics and enter the body. When they discover potentially harmful organisms or toxins, they lock onto them in an attempt to break apart and rid them from the body before they penetrate any further.

Between the probiotics and immune cells, we have a 'drag net' of sorts within the oral and nasal cavities. Should the pathogens get by the mucous, cilia, probiotics, immunoglobulins and B-cells in the mucosal membranes, and they invade tissues and cells, the immune system can switch to the cell-mediated immune strategy of attacking pathogens. This system, remember, utilizes T-cells to identify cells and tissues that have been damaged by invaders. Once the cells are identified, the T-cells utilize cytokines to signal the launch of an immune response. This involves natural killer cells (NK-cells), cytotoxic T-cells and others. Support systems include a variety of cytokine signalling devices, leucotrienes, prostaglandins and others to pump blood in, block infection, stop bleeding and begin the repair process. Around the oral cavity, this translates to redness, pain and inflammation, which often translates to a sore throat.

This cell-mediated response can also result in the launching of helper T-cells in the form of Th1 or Th2. An imbalance of Th1 to Th2 usually accompanies an allergic response, accompanied by the release of histamine. This in turn leads to a swelling of nasal passages and the throat, leading to stuffy nose and sneezing. This often leads to allergy and cold symptoms, as the body works to rebalance or control an overgrowth of fungi, bacteria and/or viruses.

In a healthy body, all of these immune responses within the mouth and nasal cavity are mediated and moderated by trillions of probiotic bacteria that line our mouth, nasal passages and our throat. Hopefully at the end of the conflict, probiotic colonies will be left in control, as their populations outnumber the pathogenic microorganisms.

Stimulating the Oral Immune System

Under the tongue are salivary glands. They produce amylase. Amylase is an enzyme that breaks down starches into simple sugars. This is one reason the body is driven to eat starches. Taking our time and chewing a little more liquefies our food and mixes them with important mucus and enzymes. Chewing well also works our jaw and face muscles. The mouth contains several parotid glands, located in the jaw behind the ears. As we chew, the parotid glands are stimulated, releasing B-cells and T-cells into the blood, mucous and lymphatic pathways. This stimulates the immune system to guard against invaders that break through the drag net.

It is also helpful to drink fewer liquids during mealtime. This allows our mucous/saliva, amylase, probiotics and immune cells to mix well with the food, damaging or destroying microorganisms before they can enter our internal tissues. Drinking too many liquids while we eat dilutes our enzymes and our probiotics. These of course assist in breaking down the molecular structure of our foods, and help block pathogen entry. A sip of room temperature water now and again to rinse the palate is more than sufficient.

Digestive Immunity

The esophagus is the staging area for food. If the mouth masticates the food well enough, the food will pass through the esophagus to the stomach within ten seconds. At the bottom of the esophagus is a valve called the esophageal sphincter. This valve lets food into the main stomach while keeping acid and food from backing up into the esophagus. An unhealthy sphincter does not close tightly enough—causing heartburn as acids and food irritate the sensitive mucous membranes of the esophagus. If the food delivered to the sphincter comes in too fast and rough, the cricopharygeus muscle, which controls the sphincter, will weaken. When this muscle loses tone, the valve weakens. This allows the stomach's acids to leak back up the esophagus, and microorganisms to leak into the stomach.

This is not the only cause for what is called heartburn. As food is dropped into the stomach, it undergoes intense churning and breakdown by the stomach's digestive juices. Special glands called gastric cells secrete a mixture of biochemicals within the stomach.

This blend is composed primarily of hydrochloric acid, pepsin, rennin and special mucus made primarily of mucopolysaccharides. De-pending upon the health of the stomach, these cells also secrete lipase, a fat-splitting enzyme. The enzymes pepsin and rennin break down proteins, preparing them for intestinal assimilation.

Gastric juice must have a particular pH to be effective. The pH is its action potential to break apart the biochemical bonds that hold together the food molecules. This means the ionic nature of our gastric juices will interfere with the biochemical bonds of the food molecules just enough to break apart those molecules into essential portions. Healthy gastric acidity will have this same effect upon any remaining microorganisms that make it through to the stomach. These very ions create an inhospitable environment for microorganisms.

In order to affect this, the acidity of gastric juice must be precise. In a healthy body, this ranges from a pH of one to three. Hydrochloric acid (HCL) is the central molecular component to reach this pH range. An acidic pH is critical to sterilize our food as well. Without enough HCL, the body runs the risk of allowing unwanted bacteria to grow in the stomach and intestines. This includes the pervasive *Helicobacter pylori* bacteria. Recent research has linked a majority of ulcers to *H. pylori* overgrowth in the stomach.

The common premise is that heartburn means too much acid in the stomach. Western medicine's solutions are antacids and acid-blockers. These will only provide a short fix for some—those with poor mucous membranes. Antacids may also create other problems, however. Antacids may also make matters worse, because they will push the pH too high. When the pH is too high, the antimicrobial quality of our stomach's acidity will be reduced, allowing the overgrowth of bacteria such as *H. pylori.*

Acid-blocking medications may further exasperate the problem in many cases. These may be helpful for temporarily easing pain and removing the symptoms, they also can create the reduction of the very digestive juices needed to break down foods for intestinal absorption. They also cut back HCL production, again allowing bacteria the ability to colonize.

Research over two decades has confirmed that more than three-quarters of ulcers involve the *Helicobacter pylori* infection. The *H. pylori* bacteria will attach and burrow into the gastric cells, eventually creating a wound in the stomach wall. For this reason, now many ulcer treatments begin with antibiotics in an attempt to kill off *H. pylori* bacteria.

Interestingly, worldwide *H. pylori* infections are much greater than ulcer levels. In many countries—especially in Africa—*H. pylori* infection rates are well above 50% of the population, yet only a small percentage of these experience ulcers. This means that there are other components to consider. Put simply: Sufficient stomach acidity and good oral probiotic populations will help protect against the overgrowth of ulcerative *H. pylori* bacteria.

In addition, special glands in the stomach called pyloric mucous glands produce and secrete a thick mucus which will provide a lining and covering for the stomach fundus, protecting it from the enzymes and acids released by the gastric pits. These mucous glands are stimulated by the vagus nerve as we begin to eat. This mucus lines the stomach cells, buffering them from the harsh gastric juices. Heartburn is often the result of too little mucus lining within the stomach and the lower esophagus. Because this lining is mostly water, those who do not drink enough water often have thin stomach mucosal linings.

Drinking water on an empty stomach improves absorption and increases the health of the mucous membranes of the entire upper digestive tract and upper respiratory tract. One of the best times to drink water is first thing in the morning before we eat and before we brush our teeth. Drinking on any empty stomach will hydrate the body faster—as the stomach directly assimilates water into the bloodstream. It will also deliver mucus from the mouth and esophagus into the stomach. To increase stomach mucus, we might consider sucking on a little sour fruit or pressing our tongue around the mouth to produce more saliva. Then we can swallow that with or without water. Doing this prior to a meal will increase our stomach mucus. Note that water should precede the meal by at least 15-20 minutes to allow for absorption. It also helps to relax and breathe prior to and during a meal. This relaxes the vagus nerve, stimulating more mucus formation. When the body is stressed, the body's activities will be drawn away from digestion, leaving the stomach with too little mucus. It is for this reason that people with too much stress will often also have heartburn.

Immune Colonization

To illustrate the general immune effects of probiotics, let's consider the increasing emergence of foodborne *Escherichia coli* outbreaks. Few of us realize that *E. coli* is a resident organism living all around us and within our guts. In a healthy body, *E. coli* colonies are heavily outnumbered by colonies of probiotics such as *Lactobacillus acidophilus* and *Bifidus regularis*, however. These probiotic colonies keep *E. coli* numbers minimized. Should new *E. coli* colonies arrive; probiotics mobilize natural antibiotics to squash and limit the invasion.

We consume *E. coli* everyday in so many foods. When we consider how few people get sick, when hundreds of thousands of people have eaten an infected food, we can see how strong of a role probiotic colonization has. Otherwise, how could such a small percentage of the thousands of people who ate a food infected with *E. coli* have gotten sick?

Furthermore, of those hundreds that may get sick from a massive *E. coli* outbreak, even fewer people actually become fatally sick: Very few people will die from a massive *E. coli* outbreak. Why? Can it simply be explained by saying that some have stronger immune systems than others?

The decisive factor is the population and composition of the body's probiotic colonies. The quantity and content of our probiotic populations make the difference between those who are easily sickened and overwhelmed by viral, bacterial or fungal infections.

Illustrating this, *Lactobacillus rhamnosus* GG or a placebo was given to 235 children hospitalized with persistent diarrhea in a randomized, double-blind and controlled study in India (Basu *et al.* 2007). *Escherichia coli* were the most common bacteria infecting the children, followed by *Shigella* spp. and *Clostridium difficile*. The average illness duration was significantly lower among the probiotic group (5.3 days versus 9.2 days), and the average hospital stay was also significantly less among the probiotic group.

In other words, those with healthy probiotic populations will have stronger immunity against infection and foodborne illnesses. In fact, our bodies typically already contain *E. coli* and *Salmonella* bacteria. Several strains of *E. coli* will often reside in a healthy intestinal tract. These do not make us sick because our probiotic bacteria populations keep *E. coli* populations from growing too large. As we've discussed, probiotics produce their own array of antibiotic substances, which inhibit or control pathogenic microorganism populations. The table below summarizes the results of two laboratory studies and a review of the research (Chaitow and

Trenev 1990) measuring the inhibition zone (or killing distance) three probiotics have upon selected pathogenic bacteria:

Bacteria Inhibition by Selected Probiotics

Pathogen	L. acidophilus[1]	L. bulgaricus[2]	B. bifidum[3]
Escherichia coli	44mm	40mm	20mm
Clostridium botulinum	37mm	38mm	not tested
Clostridium perfringens	31mm	33mm	not tested
Proteus mirabilis	39mm	45mm	not tested
Salmonella enteridis	42mm	39mm	not tested
Salmonella typhimurium	44mm	39mm	not tested
Salmonella typhosa	not tested	not tested	12mm
Shigella dysenteriae	30mm	not tested	11mm
Shigella paradysenteriae	30mm	not tested	not tested
Staphylococcus aureus	35mm	38mm	23mm
Staphylococcus faecalis	31mm	39mm	not tested
Bacillus cereus	not tested	not tested	22mm
Pseudomonas fluorescens	not tested	not tested	18mm
Mocrococcus flavis	not tested	not tested	25mm

1. Laboratory tests on *Lactobacillus acidophilus* secretion acidophilin DDS1 adapted from Fernandes *et al.* 1988.
2. Laboratory tests on *Lactobacillus* bulgaricus DDS14 secretion bulgarican adapted from Fernandes *et al.* 1988.
3. Laboratory tests on *Bifidobacterium bifidum* 1452 adapted from Anand *et al.* 1984.

This illustrates that, like animals within a forest, bacteria colonies balance and control each other's populations. In a healthy body well-colonized with probiotic populations, our bodies harbor enough probiotics with their own 'smart' antibacterial strategies to keep most bacteria from overgrowth.

The same goes for the oral and nasal cavities. A healthy upper respiratory tract and upper digestive tract will contain a balance of strong probiotic colonies that control intruding and resident species.

The Probiotic Gatekeepers

The human body houses huge populations of living bacteria forms. About one hundred trillion bacteria live in the body's digestive system—about 3.5 pounds worth. The upper respiratory tract and digestive tract contains about 700 different bacteria and fungi species. About twenty species make up about 75% of the population, however. Many of these are our resident strains, which attach to our mucosal membranes and intestinal walls. Other probiotic strains are transient. These transient strains will typically stay for no more than about 12 days.

Microorganisms living within our bodies may be probiotic, pathobiotic or eubiotic. A probiotic is a microorganism living within the body while contributing positively to the body's health. These friendly bacteria also are also called flora—meaning "healthful." The pathobiotic is a microorganism that harms or impedes the body in one way or another. Eubiotics can be either harmful or helpful to the body, depending upon their colony size and location. A healthy body contains a substantially greater number of probiotics than pathobiotics, while a diseased body likely contains more pathobiotic than probiotic populations.

One haunting question in this discussion is how many pathobiotics are actually eubiotics. In other words, how many disease-causing bacteria are actually normal or occasional residents in a healthy body that simply have gotten out of control? Quite a few, according to the research.

Again, probiotics line mucosal linings around our oral cavity, gums, teeth, nasal cavity, throat, esophagus, and associated membranes. These probiotics deter the entry of pathogenic bacteria, viruses and fungi through the mouth and nose. Assuming the colonies are strong enough, even if the immune system is not able to properly identify or attack the invader, the oral probiotic system will remove the invader in short order. This will be accomplished by the probiotics producing certain acids and antibiotics that either specifically kill that type of invader or create an environment within which the invader does not feel comfortable.

Oral probiotics will vigorously defend the gums and teeth. They will attach to and inhabit the spaces between our gums and our teeth. The problem arises when our diets become overly sugary. As we will discuss later in more detail, probiotics require complex oligosaccharides like inulin, FOS (fructooligosaccharides) and GOS (galactooligosaccharides) for food sources. They do not thrive from simple sugars like glucose and sucrose. Pathogenic bacteria, on the other hand, typically thrive from these simple sugars. In fact, they can grow quite quickly, and may immediately begin to outnumber the probiotic populations. As they do this, they secrete acids that damage our teeth and infect our gums.

The upper respiratory tract and digestive systems are not the only places probiotics guard against invaders and maintain healthy tissues. The vagina, the skin, the urinary tract and the anus are also inhabited by species of probiotics that guard against intrusion. Healthy colonies of these species protect us against pathogens and toxins, and support healthy tissues.

Within the intestines, probiotics attach to and dwell in between the villi and microvilli. This prevents pathogenic bacteria from infecting those cells. Probiotics also break down foods and monitor the food molecules being presented to the intestinal wall for absorption. This helps prevent the body from absorbing molecules that are too large or not sufficiently broken down. As we will discuss further, large, atypical food molecules that have entered the bloodstream will stimulate an inflammatory and allergic response, often in the sinuses. This is because these larger molecules are not recognized by the immune system.

This is often the case with wheat proteins, milk proteins and nut proteins. For many people, they will be able to drink milk or eat nuts or breads for many years. Then suddenly they become allergic or sensitive to one or a number of them. Why? Larger proteins from these foods are being allowed into the bloodstream.

Our probiotic colonies keep down pathogens while protecting our bodies from the endotoxins produced by pathogenic bacteria and fungi. In an imbalanced body, these endotoxins are often absorbed into the bloodstream through the gums, the intestinal walls and/or through the colon. Once inside the bloodstream, these endotoxins may be absorbed into organs and cells. This gives rise to inflammation and pain as the body works to purge these toxins.

These facts, together with the research showing probiotic supplements ease many autoimmune symptoms; surely give us good reason to suspect that many autoimmune diseases may actually be caused by imbalances between our probiotics and pathogenic microorganisms.

Probiotic Inoculation

Our body establishes its resident strains during the first year to eighteen months. Our first major encounter with large populations of probiotic bacteria comes when our baby body descends the cervix and emerges from the vagina. During this birthing journey—assuming a healthy mother—we are exposed to numerous species of future resident probiotics. This first inoculation provides an advanced immune shield to keep populations of pathobiotics at bay.

Because we get much of our bacteria as we pass through the vagina, Caesarean section babies have been shown to carry significantly lower colonies of healthy bacteria. *Bifidobacterium infantis* is considered the healthiest probiotic colonizing infants. Research has indicated that while 60% of vagina-birth babies have *B. infantis* colonies, only 9% of C-section babies are colonized with probiotics, and only 9% of those are colonized with *B. infantis.* This means that less than one percent of C-section babies are properly colonized with *B. infantis,* while 60% of vagina births are colonized with *B. infantis.*

Following the inoculation from the vagina, further colonization is accomplished from a combination of breast-feeding and putting everything in our mouths, from our parent's fingers to anything we find as we are crawling around the ground. These activities can provide a host of different bacteria—both pathobiotic and probiotic.

Mother's colostrum (early milk) may contain up to 40% probiotics by volume. This will be abundant in bifidobacteria and probiotic streptococci, assuming the mother is not taking antibiotics. Healthy strains of bifidobacteria and streptococci typically colonize our body first and set up an environment for other groups of bacteria, such as lactobacilli, to become established.

Picking up a good mix of cooperative probiotic residents is a crucial part of the establishment of our body's immune system. Many of the probiotic strains we inherit from our mothers as infants become permanent residents. They will continue the same duties they had within mama, to protect against infection by lining the body's various mucosal membranes while stimulating our immune systems.

Gaining early probiotic strains from the environment may appear difficult to understand, as we have been taught that dirt is infectious. Rather, natural soils contain huge populations of various bacteria. Many of these are spore-forming *soil-based organisms.* Some soil-based organisms or SBOs can become probiotic populations after early ingestion. Others, which may be less healthy to the body, will allow exposure to probiotic colonies and the immune system to counteract those strains in the future. This training mechanism is critical to the body's future immunity. This means those important infantile occupations—crawling on all fours, eating dirt, making mud pies, having food fights, playing tag and so on—all come together to deliver a stronger immune system later in life.

This has been confirmed by recent research illustrating that infants raised in sterile environments are more likely to suffer from allergies, infections and food sensitivities. Parents should consider living in a natural setting or at least outings to natural environments like pesticide free parks to provide exposure to pathogens and future probiotic colonies.

Housing the Resident Strains

As these early probiotics set up shop within our mouths, intestines and elsewhere, they become recognized by the body's immune system. They also become incubated in parts of the body's lymphatic system. The vermiform appendix, for example, was observed in 2007 by scientists at Duke University (Randal, *et al.*) as housing resident probiotic strains, and releasing them into the cecum during increased infection. It seems that finally the purpose for the mysterious appendix has been discovered after decades of surgical removal. There is good reason to believe that other lymph duct centers such as the tonsils may also incubate resident probiotic strains.

Indeed, the delivery of probiotics with mother's breast milk indicates that probiotics have a pathway and route of residence within the mammary glands, which are fed by the lymphatic system. This indicates that resident probiotic bacteria move within the lymphatic system. Just as mother delivers various immunoglobulins from the immune system via breast milk, she also delivers probiotics through similar pathways.

We can house many transient probiotics at any particular time, but our resident probiotic bacteria strains do not change through adulthood. Once they take up residence, those strains become part of our body's ecosystem. This does not mean they always remain in strong numbers. Over years of stress, antibiotics and toxin exposure, resident strains may become dramatically reduced, and possibly even eliminated. This is logical, as dramatic immunosuppressive states and issues such as fibromyalgia often follow periods of extended antibiotic use.

Supplemented probiotics do not appear to replace these resident strains. Supplemented probiotics typically remain for a couple of weeks, more or less, depending upon the strain and our internal environment. It is believed by some experts that with continued dosing of supplemental strains, resident strains—if they are still present—may regrow in colony strength.

Illustrating strain-specific survival among children, Polish scientists (Szymański *et al.* 2006) gave *Lactobacillus rhamnosus* to children with diarrhea. The researchers found that some *L. rhamnosus* strains given were found among 80% of patients after 5 days, and among 41.3% after 14 days. One particular strain, *L. rhamnosus* 573L/1, *"colonized the G.I. tract more persistently,"* according to the researchers.

Territorial Behavior

Some of our bacteria live peacefully together. Most struggle with other colonies, and mark clearly defined territories with special biochemical secretions. Probiotics within the same colony usually specialize in particular functions. Some work together to help break down foods, and some guard and protect their territory as they consume metabolites. To protect against pathogens, most will produce a number of natural antibiotics designed to reduce their competitor populations. At the same time, their antibiotic secretions aid the body's immune system by stimulating T-cell and B-cell activity.

Many probiotics release antibiotic secretions called bacteriocins that selectively reduce the growth of other pathogens, including yeasts and pathobiotics. In other words, their antibiotic secretions—unlike many pharmaceutical antibiotics—can selectively damage certain strains of microorganisms and not others. Probiotics can produce lactic acid, acetic acid, hydrogen peroxide, lactoperoxidase, lipopolysaccharides, and a number of other antibacterial substances. Lactic acid, for example, helps acidify the intestines and prevent harmful bacteria overgrowth.

To give an idea of just how diligent and efficient probiotic bacteria are in producing antibacterial components, a study at the Department of Microbiology of the Abaseheb Garware College in India (Watve *et al.* 2001) studied the genus *Steptomyces* since the 1970s, and found that it has been producing new antibiotic substances exponentially over the years. They statistically graphed the count of antimicrobial substances produced over the years, and estimated that the genus has likely produced more than 100,000 different antibiotic compounds over that period!

Because bacteria are living organisms, they are *adaptable.* This means that they will respond to new competition with new antibiotic tools. They will produce different types of biochemicals, and develop different means of attack.

Most bacteria also manufacture waste products. Some of these are toxic and some of them are beneficial. Pathobiotics manufacture substances that increase the risk of disease by raising the body's toxicity level in addition to infecting cells. Various immunological diseases directly or indirectly stem from the waste streams of pathobiotics. Harmful bacteria can overload the liver and lymph systems with toxins. The toxins produced by bacteria are referred to as endotoxins—a technical name for bacteria poop. Bacteria defecate just as any other living organism does. Endotoxins from pathogenic bacteria can contribute to or directly stimulate inflammation and irritation within and around the gums, the nasal cavity and the throat.

Increased risks of cardiovascular diseases such as atherosclerosis and stroke have been connected to periodontal disease over the past decade of research. The mechanism is currently unknown, but there is suspicion that the NF-kappa signalling system appears to be stimulated by periodontal bacteria. As NF-kappa is associated with other toxic or free radical exposures, it is likely that the stimulating factor is the endotoxin output by these bacteria. As we've discussed, bacteria endotoxins stimulate inflammation because they are, well, toxic.

Illustrating this, Finnish scientists (Isolauri *et al.* 1994) gave lactobacilli probiotics to 42 children with acute rotavirus diarrhea. They found that the probiotics significantly reduced levels of the bacterial endotoxin urease, and lessened infection duration among the probiotic group compared to the placebo group.

It only makes sense to assure that our bacteria populations anywhere in our body—including our mouths, throats and nasal cavities—are in balance. Balance means that our probiotic bacteria significantly outnumber and control pathogenic microorganisms. Let's explore some of the diseases that are specifically related to this balance of microorganisms.

Oral Probiotics and Disease

Science is still unfolding the complex mechanisms and many benefits derived from the more than 700 species of still largely unresearched microorganisms that inhabit our bodies from head to toe with vast populations concentrated in our mouths and intestines.

Summary of Probiotic Mechanisms

In *Probiotics - Protection Against Infection: Using Nature's Tiny Warriors to Stem Infection and Fight Disease* (Adams 2009), we reviewed over 600 human clinical studies and cited more than 450 studies and reports to conclude a host of general immune system effects from primarily ingested probiotics. While we cite these same studies in the reference section of this book, the aforementioned book specifically details each of the effects listed below.

This table summarizes the results from randomized, double-blinded (or at least blinded), and placebo-controlled human clinical studies on the effects of probiotics in the human body:

Allergies	reduce Th1/ Th2 ratio; decrease Th2 levels; lower TGF-beta2; increase IgE
Anorexia nervosa	increase appetite; increase assimilation; increase lymphocytes
antibiotics	produce antibiotic and antifungal substances (such as acidophillin and bifidin) that repel or kill pathogenic bacteria, adjusting to pathogen and resistance
B-cells	modulate and redirect B-cell activity
Bile	break down bile acids
Biochemicals	secrete lactic acids, lactoperoxidases, formic acids, lipopolysaccharides, peptidoglycans, superantigens and others to manage pH and repel pathogens.
Bladder cancer	reduce recurrent bladder cancer incidence and inhibit new tumors
Blood pressure	reduce hypertension; inhibit ACE
Calcium	increase serum calcium; decrease parathyroid hormone
Cancer (general)	reduce mutagenicity; increase natural killer tumoricidal activity; increase survival rates

Candida overgrowth	control populations; reduce overgrowths
CD cell orientation	modulate and direct particular CD cells depending upon condition, including CD56, CD8, CD4, CD25, CD69, CD2, others
Cell degeneration	slow cellular degeneration and associated diseases among elderly persons
Colds and Influenza	reduce infection frequency; reduce infection duration; reduce symptoms; prevent complications; decrease worker sick days
Colic	reduce crying time; decrease infection; increase stool frequency; decrease bloating and indigestion
Colon cancer	reduce recurrence; increase survival rates; reduce beta-glucosidase; inhibit cell abnormality and mutation; increase IL-2
Constipation	increase bowel movement frequency; ease colon and impacted feces
Control pathogens	compete with pathogenic organisms for nutrients, thus checking their growth
C-reactive protein	reduce levels in blood
Cytokines	stimulate the body's production of various cytokines, including IL-6, IL-3, IL-5, TNF alpha, and interferon
Dental caries	reduce and control cavity-causing bacteria
Digestion	reduce gas, nausea and stress-related gastrointestinal digestive difficulty
Digestive difficulty	secrete digestive enzymes; help break down nutrients from fats; proteins and other foods
Diverticulosis	reduce polyps and strengthen intestinal wall mucosa
Ear infections	hasten otitis media healing response; prevent infections
EFAs	manufacture essential fatty acids, including important short-chained fatty acids, and help the body assimilate EFAs
Fiber digestion	aid in soluble fiber fermentation, yielding fatty acids and energy
Food poisoning	increase resistance to food poisoning; battle and remove pathogenic organisms; reduce diarrhea and other symptoms
Glucose metabolism	improve glucose control
Gum disease	reduce gum infections; deplete gingivitis
H. pylori	reduce H. pylori infections; reduce ulcers
HIV/AIDS	stimulate immune system; reduce symptoms;

	reduce co-infections; increase survival rates
Hormones	balance and stimulate hormone production
Hydrogen peroxide	manufacture H2O2 - oxygenating/antiseptic
IBS	decrease bloating, pain, cramping
Immunoglobulins	modulate IgA, IgG, IgE, IgM to weakness
Inflammation	modify prostaglandins (E1, E2), IFN-gamma, reduce CRP; modulate TNF-alpha; increase IgA; slow inflammatory response as needed
Intestinal Permeability	protect against IIPS; block penetration of toxins; work cooperatively with villi and microvilli; attach to mucosa; improve barrier function
Intestine walls	protect walls of intestines against toxin exposure and colonization of pathogens
Iron absorption	increase iron assimilation; increase hemoglobin count
Keratoconjunctivitis	decrease burning, itching and dry eyes
Kidney stones	reduce urine oxalates; reduce blood oxalates
Lipids/Cholesterol	reduce LDL, triglycerides and total cholesterol; increase HDL
Liver	stimulate liver cells (hepatocytes); stimulate liver function; reduce cirrhosis symptoms; reduce liver enzymes
Liver cancer	stimulate immune response; decrease infection and complications after surgery
Lung cancer	increase survival rates; reduce chest pain and other symptoms
Mental state	improve mood; stimulate positive mood hormones like serotonin and tryptophan
Milk digestion	aid dairy digestion for lactose-intolerant people; produce lactase
Monocytes	increase oxidative burst capacity
Mucosa	coat intestines, stomach, oral, nasal and vagina mucosa, providing protective barrier
NF-kappaB	modulate activity to condition
NK-cells	stimulate natural killer cell activity
Nutrition	manufacture biotin, thiamin (B1), riboflavin (B2), niacin (B3), pantothenic acid (B5), pyridoxine (B6), cobalamine (B12), folic acid, vitamin A and/or vitamin K; aid in assimilation of proteins, fats and minerals
Pancreatitis	reduce pancreas infection (sepsis); reduce necrosis; speed healing
pH control	produce a number of other acids and biochemicals, modulating pH (see biochemicals)

Phagocytes	increase phagocytic activity as needed
Phytonutrients	convert to bioavailable nutrient forms
Premature births and Low birth weights	speed growth; reduce infection; improve immune response; increase nutrition
Protein assimilation	break down amino acid content; inhibit assimilation of allergic polypeptides
Respiratory infections	inhibit pneumonia; reduce duration of infection; inhibit bronchitis; inhibit tonsillitis
Rotavirus infections	speed healing times; prevent infection; ease abdominal pain; eradicate infective agents
Spleen	stimulate spleen activity
Stomach cancer	inhibit tumors; reduce *H. pylori* overgrowths
T-cells	modulate T-cell activity to condition
Th1 - Th2	decrease Th2 activity; increase Th1 (increases healing and decreases allergic response)
Thymus	increase thymus size and activity
Toxins	break down toxins; inhibit assimilation of heavy metals, chemicals, and endotoxins
Ulcers	control *H. pylori*; speed healing; improve mucosa; moderate acids; reduce pain
Vaccination	increase vaccine effectiveness
Vaginosis/Vaginitis	reduce infection; re-establish healthy pH; reduce odor

Amazingly, this is not even a complete list of all the probiotic effects found in human clinical research. Furthermore, medical researchers have only chosen a small portion of probiotics' possible health benefits for controlled human research. In other words, the research is only beginning.

Oral Cavity Probiotic Research

Here we will review a sampling of the research on oral or intestinal probiotics for a number of human disease pathologies. These relate either to the upper respiratory tract, ears, skin and other areas not typically related to probiotics. Much of the research we discuss here utilized probiotic lozenges, gums or chewable tablets. Other studies document upper respiratory tract effects utilizing intestinal probiotics. The latter indicate that even though ingested supplemental probiotics temporarily colonize the intestines, they will still affect pathologies of the upper respiratory tract. For a wider range of effects from intestinal probiotics, see the author's book, *Probiotics - Protection Against Infection* (2009).

Whether mentioned here or not, practically every study reviewed below was a randomized, placebo-controlled and double-blinded or at least blinded study. Furthermore, all were done by reputable scientists and published in peer-reviewed journals. In most cases, the strain detail is included in our review. This does not necessarily mean that the effects of that species are limited to the particular strain being identified. Over the history of research on probiotics, there have been many common effects among different strains of the same species. This is not universal, however. Many strains have been shown to be more effective or stronger in their actions than other strains of the same species. We'll discuss this further in the supplement section.

Periodontal Disease and Dental Caries

The gums and teeth are coated with legions of different bacteria—some probiotic and some pathogenic. Typical oral bacteria include *Streptococcus mutans, Streptococcus salivarius, Lactobacillus salivarius, E. coli, Streptococcus pyogenes, Porphyromonas gingivalis, Tannerella forsynthensis,* and *Prevotella intermedia.* With a diet containing too many simple sugars and poor dental hygiene, the pathogenic bacteria can overwhelm the probiotics, causing infected gums. As pathogenic populations of *S. mutans, S. pyogenes, P. gingivalis, T. forsynthensis* and *P. intermedia* come into greater numbers, serious infections can occur. These conditions are often symptomized by gingivitis, tooth root infection, jawbone infections and general periodontal disease.

Streptococcus mutans was first isolated in 1924, but it was not linked to dental caries until the early 1960s. *S. mutans* and other cavity-forming bacteria consume sugars and carbohydrates from our foods, and produce destructive acids such as lactic acid. These acids interact with the calcium in tooth enamel, forming plaque. This interaction and plaque-formation creates cavities—dental caries.

This has led most researchers to consider *Streptococcus mutans* a eubiotic: a probiotic or non-pathogenic at controlled colony sizes. Like many other eubiotic yeasts and bacteria, it is a natural resident of the mouth that can easily grow beyond its healthy population size due to imbalances in the diet and oral hygiene.

A number of studies have confirmed that *Streptococcus mutans* tends to pass from mother to child. Therefore, it makes sense for mothers to control these populations to avoid passing them on to their children.

All of the bacteria mentioned above and others can reside in both healthy and infected mouths. The strategy promoted by the modern medical and dental industries is to try to kill virtually all bacteria with various antiseptic mouthwashes and toothpastes. As we can see from continuing statistics on gingivitis and dental caries, these strategies are not working very well. A better strategy may be to use nature's probiotic populations to create a balance between the healthy bacteria and the disease-promoting bacteria. If probiotic populations are maximized, they will deplete and manage the pathogenic bacteria populations.

Let's see how this is supported by the research:

Researchers from the Istanbul's Yeditepe University Dental School conducted a number of studies on periodontal disease using *Lactobacillus reuteri* ATCC 55730 and *Bifidobacterium lactis*.

The researchers (Caglar *et al.* 2006) gave *Lactobacillus reuteri* ATCC 55730 or placebo to 120 young adults through straw or lozenge daily for 3 weeks. Before and after treatment, colony populations of the periodontal disease culprit *Streptococcus mutans* were measured. After the treatment period, *Streptococcus mutans* populations were significantly reduced among the probiotic groups as compared to the placebo group. *S. mutans* levels were also significantly lower compared to before treatment among the probiotic groups.

A year later, the researchers (Caglar *et al.* 2007) gave placebo or *Lactobacillus reuteri* probiotic chewing gums to 80 healthy young adults three times daily for three weeks. Those given the *L. reuteri* gum had significantly reduced levels of oral *Streptococcus mutans* compared to placebo and before treatment.

The researchers (Caglar *et al.* 2008) then gave 24 healthy young adult volunteers ice-cream containing *Bifidobacterium lactis* Bb-12 or a placebo ice cream for 40 days. Once again, oral *Streptococcus mutans* counts were significantly reduced in the probiotic ice cream group compared to the placebo group and compared to before treatment.

The researchers (Caglar *et al.* 2008) then gave oral lozenges of *Lactobacillus reuteri* or a placebo to 20 healthy young women: half received the *L. reuteri* and half received the placebo lozenge. After sucking on one lozenge a day for 10 days through a specially devised medical device, oral pathogen *Streptococcus mutans* levels were significantly reduced among the probiotic group, compared to the placebo group. Again, *S. mutans* levels were significantly lower among the probiotic group and compared to levels existing prior to treatment.

Other research has arrived at similar results. Scientists from Italy's University of L'Aquila, Department of Experimental Medicine (Riccia *et al.* 2007) gave 8 healthy volunteers and 21 chronic periodontitis patients *Lactobacillus brevis* lozenges. The probiotic treatment led to the total disappearance of all clinical symptoms among the subjects. Probiotic treatment also resulted in a significant decrease in gum inflammatory markers such as nitrite/nitrate, PGE2, matrix metalloproteinase, and saliva IFN-gamma.

Researchers at Japan's Tohoku University Graduate School of Dentistry (Shimauchi *et al.* 2008) treated 66 human volunteers with freeze-dried *Lactobacillus salivarius* WB21 lozenge tablets or a placebo for 8 weeks. Periodontal testing following the eight weeks confirmed that the probiotic group had significantly greater improvements in plaque index and probing pocket depth compared to the placebo group and before treatment.

Scientists from the University of Copenhagen (Twetman *et al.* 2009) gave three groups either chewing gum with placebo or two strains of *Lactobacillus reuteri* for 10 minutes a day for two weeks. Their gums were examined and given immunoassays for gingivitis inflammation. Bleeding on probing was significantly less among the probiotic groups. TNF-alpha and IL-8 significantly decreased among the probiotic subjects. IL-1beta also decreased during the chewing period. The researchers concluded that, *"The reduction of pro-inflammatory cytokines in GCF may be proof of principle for the probiotic approach combating inflammation in the oral cavity."*

Researchers from the Institute of Dentistry at the University of Helsinki (Näse *et al.* 2001) investigated the effect of *Lactobacillus rhamnosus* GG on dental caries. Milk with or without *Lactobacillus rhamnosus* GG was given to 594 children ages 1 to 6 years old. The probiotic group had significantly less dental caries and significantly lower *S. mutans* counts by the end of the study—especially among the 3- to 4-year-olds.

Scientists from the Universidad Nacional Autónoma de Mexico (Bayona *et al.* 1990) gave 245 seven-year-old children chewable tablets of either pyridoxine (vitamin B6) with heat-killed probiotics (streptococci and lactobacilli) or tablets with pyridoxine once a week for 16 weeks. Four evaluations were made over a two-year period from the beginning of the study. There was a 42% reduction of dental caries among the probiotic group compared to the placebo group of children.

Scientists from Sweden's Malmö University (Krasse *et al.* 2006) gave *Lactobacillus reuteri* or placebo to 59 patients with moderate to severe gingivitis. After 2 weeks of treatment, the gingival index and plaque index were established from measurements of two teeth surfaces and from saliva. The average gingival index and plaque index was significantly lower in the *L. reuteri* probiotic groups. The researchers concluded that, *"Lactobacillus reuteri was efficacious in reducing both gingivitis and plaque in patients with moderate to severe gingivitis."*

Finnish researchers from the University of Helsinki (Ahola *et al.* 2002) found that the long-term consumption of milk containing *Lactobacillus rhamnosus* GG significantly reduced dental caries. They also found this same effect resulted from probiotic cheese ingestion. To illustrate this later effect, the researchers gave 74 young adults a placebo or 60 grams of probiotic cheese per day for three weeks. There were significantly lower salivary *Streptococcus mutans* counts among the probiotic cheese group.

Italian scientists (Petti *et al.* 2001) gave healthy volunteers either yogurt with *Streptococcus thermophilus* and *Lactobacillus bulgaricus* or non-probiotic ice cream for 8 weeks. The probiotic group had lower levels of salivary *Streptococcus mutans* than the control group. However, *L. bulgaricus* was only transiently detected in the oral cavity, indicating that it did not colonize well within the mouth, contrasting with other research on species such as *Lactobacillus reuteri* and *Streptococcus salivarius*.

Florida researcher gave a mouthwash containing *Streptococcus oralis* KJ3, *Streptococcus uberis* KJ2, and *Streptococcus rattus* to a small group of children twice daily for four weeks. After the period, the mouthwash significantly reduced the levels of *S. mutans* and other pathogenic bacteria among the children's teeth.

Other probiotics are also antagonistic to *S. mutans.* In 2010, Dr. Christine Lang, a German researcher presented findings at the International Probiotics Association World Congress that after screening 700 Lactobacillus strains, they found six strains that bind to S. mutans. Binding to the bacteria means decreasing its attachment to gums and teeth and reducing its damaging effects.

Of these six, *Lactobacillus paracasei* had the greatest binding ability.

Bacterial Infections

We have already discussed how probiotics can conquer and re-duce colonies of a multitude of bacteria. This occurs as a result of probiotics producing a number of antibiotic substances, along with acidic biochemicals. As a result, probiotics have been shown to reduce the incidence of strep throat, tonsillitis, *E. coli* infections, mastitis, burn infections and many others. Here are a few studies illustrating these effects:

Researchers from New Zealand's University of Otago (Dierksen *et al.* 2007) gave 219 children milk supplemented with *Strepto-coccus salivarius* K12 for either 2 days or 9 days. At the beginning of the treatment, a significant number of the children had higher levels of infective *Streptococcus pyrogenes* (which can lead to strep throat and necrotizing fasciitis) populations on the tongue. Follow-ing probiotic supplementation, increased levels of salivaricin (pro-duced by *Streptococcus salivarius*) was found among the probiotic group. This antibiotic substance produced by *Streptococcus salivar-ius* significantly inhibits *Streptococcus pyogenes*.

Researchers at Spain's Hospital Materno-Infantil Vall d'Hebron (Tormo *et al.* 2006) treated 35 infants with gastrointestinal prob-lems with a placebo or a probiotic blend of *Lactobacillus acidophi-lus* La5, *Bifidobacterium lactis* Bb 12, *Streptococcus thermophilus* and *Lactobacillus bulgaricus* plus prebiotic oligofructose. After one week of treatment, nasogastric aspirate testing showed that the probiotic group had significantly lower incidence of pathogenic bacteria compared to the placebo group (43% versus 75%). The probiotic group also had fewer infections of pathogenic microor-ganisms (39% versus 75%).

Scientists from the Department of Nutrition at Spain's Univer-sidad Completeness de Madrid (Jimenez *et al.* 2008) studied 20 women with staphylococcal mastitis in a randomized placebo-controlled study. The probiotic group was given *Lactobacillus sali-varius* CECT5713 and *Lactobacillus gasseri* CECT5714 (both origi-nally isolated from breast milk) for 4 weeks, and the control group was given a placebo. After 30 days, staphylococcal counts within the probiotic group were significantly lower than the control group (2.96 log(10) CFU/ml versus 4.79 log(10) CFU/ml). Furthermore, *L. salivarius* and *L. gasseri* were also isolated from the breast milk of

6 of the 10 women in the probiotic group. After 14 days of treatment, there were no clinical signs of mastitis observed within the probiotic group. Mastitis persisted among the placebo group.

Eighty burn patients from an Argentina hospital burn unit (Peral *et al.* 2009) had infected second- and third-degree burns, along with non-infected third-degree burns. They were given topical applications of probiotic *Lactobacillus plantarum* or silver sulphadiazine (SD-Ag). (SD-Ag is a typical antimicrobial paste often used to prevent burn infections. This comes with some adverse side effects however.) Among both infected and non-infected burns, *L. plantarum* prevented wound infection, and promoted wound granulation healing equal to or better than SD-Ag, without the side effects.

Researchers from the University of Paris (Schiffrin *et al.* 1997) gave 28 volunteers either *Lactobacillus acidophilus* or *Bifidobacterium bifidum* strain Bb12. Phagocytosis (killing) of *Escherichia coli* was enhanced in both probiotic groups.

Ukrainian scientists (Marushko 2000) examined 77 children with streptococcal tonsillitis. They found that the infections were symptomized by a reduction in *"tonsil colony resistance."* The study also found that *L. acidophilus* provided a *"highly efficient means of treating tonsillitis of streptococcal etiology."*

Allergies

Allergies have been increasing over the past few decades. Modern medical research is puzzled with this progression. Why are suddenly more people becoming allergic to the plants and pollens that have surrounded humans for thousands of years? This is a huge topic, but we do know from the research that the lack of healthy probiotic colonies is a major factor in our body's ability to reduce toxin levels and reduce allergic sensitivities.

Probiotics mechanisms have been increasingly connected to inflammatory and allergic responses. They play a critical role in maintaining the epithelial barrier function of the intestinal tract. Allergies appear to increase with intestinal permeability. Without an adequate intestinal barrier, larger food molecules, endotoxins and microorganisms can enter the bloodstream more easily. These increase the body's total toxin burden, making the body more sensitive to environmental inputs such as pollens and foods. Here we review some of the allergy research, which includes traditional sinus allergies as well as allergic skin responses.

Japanese scientists (Ishida *et al.* 2003) gave a drink with *Lactobacillus acidophilus* strain L-92 or a placebo to 49 patients with perennial allergic rhinitis for eight weeks. The probiotic group showed significant improvement in runny nose and watery eyes symptoms, along with decreased nasal mucosa swelling and redness compared to the placebo group. These results were also duplicated in a follow-up study (2005) of 23 allergy sufferers by some of the same researchers.

Research from Sweden's Linköping University (Böttcher *et al.* 2008) gave *Lactobacillus reuteri* or a placebo to 99 pregnant women from gestational week 36 until infant delivery. The babies were followed for two years after birth, and analyzed for eczema and allergen sensitization and immunity markers. Probiotic supplementation lowered TGF-beta2 levels in mother's milk and babies' feces and slightly increased IL-10 levels in mothers' colostrum. Lower levels of TGF-beta2 are associated with lower sensitization and lower risk of IgE-associated eczema.

German researchers (Grönlund *et al.* 2007) tested 61 infants and mother pairs for allergic status and bifidobacteria levels from 30-35 weeks of gestation and from one-month old. Every mother's breast milk contained some type of bifidobacteria, with *Bifidobacterium longum* found most frequently. However, only the infants of allergic, atopic mothers had colonization with *B. adolescentis.* Allergic mothers also had significantly less bifidobacteria in their breast-milk versus non-allergic mothers. Infants of allergic mothers also had less bifidobacteria in the feces than did infants from non-allergic mothers.

Japanese scientists (Xiao *et al.* 2006) gave 44 patients with Japanese cedar pollen allergies *Bifidobacterium longum* BB536 for 13 weeks. The probiotic group had significantly decreased symptoms of rhinorrhea (runny nose) and nasal blockage versus the placebo group. The probiotic group also had decreased activity among plasma T-helper type 2 (Th2) cells and increased activity among Japanese cedar pollen-specific IgE. The researchers concluded that the results, *"suggest the efficacy of BB536 in relieving JCPsis symptoms, probably through the modulation of Th2-skewed immune response."*

Researchers from the Wellington School of Medicine and Health Sciences at New Zealand's University of Otago (Wickens *et al.* 2008) studied the association between probiotics and eczema in 474 children. Pregnant women took either a placebo, *Lactobacil-*

lus rhamnosus HN001, or *Bifidobacterium animalis* subsp *lactis* strain HN019 starting from 35 weeks gestation, and their babies received the same treatment from birth to 2 years old. The probiotic infants given *L. rhamnosus* had significantly lower incidence of eczema compared with infants taking the placebo. There was no significant difference between the *B. animalis* group and the placebo group, however.

Researchers from Japan's Kansai Medical University Kouri Hospital (Hattori *et al.* 2003) gave 15 children with atopic dermatitis either *Bifidobacterium breve* M-16V or a placebo. After one month, the probiotic group had a significant improvement of allergic symptoms.

Researchers from Tokyo's Juntendo University School of Medicine (Fujii *et al.* 2006) gave 19 preterm infants placebo or *Bifidobacterium breve* supplementation for three weeks after birth. Anti-inflammatory serum TGF-beta1 levels in the probiotic group were elevated on day 14 and remained elevated through day 28. Messenger RNA expression was enhanced for the probiotic group on day 28 compared with the placebo group. The researchers concluded that, *"These results demonstrated that the administration of B. breve to preterm infants can up-regulate TGF-beta1 signaling and may possibly be beneficial in attenuating inflammatory and allergic reactions in these infants."*

Scientists from Britain's Institute of Food Research (Ivory *et al.* 2008) gave *Lactobacillus casei* Shirota (LcS) to 10 patients with seasonal allergic rhinitis. The researchers compared immune status with daily ingestion of a milk drink with or without live *Lactobacillus casei* over a period of 5 months. Blood samples were tested for plasma IgE and grass pollen-specific IgG by an enzyme immunoassay. Patients treated with *Lactobacillus casei* milk showed significantly reduced levels of antigen-induced IL-5, IL-6 and IFN-gamma production compared with the placebo group. Levels of specific IgG also increased and IgE decreased in the probiotic group. The researchers concluded that, *"These data show that probiotic supplementation modulates immune responses in allergic rhinitis and may have the potential to alleviate the severity of symptoms."*

Researchers from the Skin and Allergy Hospital at the University of Helsinki (Kukkonen *et al.* 2007) studied the role of probiotics and allergies with 1,223 pregnant women carrying children with a high-risk of allergies. A placebo or lactobacilli and bifidobacteria combination with GOS was given to the pregnant women for 2 to 4 weeks before delivery, and their babies continued the treatment after birth. At two years of age, the infants in the probiotic group had 25% less chance of eczema and 34% less chance of contracting atopic eczema.

The same researchers from the Skin and Allergy Hospital and Helsinki University Central Hospital (Kukkonen *et al.* 2009) studied the immune effects of feeding probiotics to pregnant mothers. 925 pregnant mothers were given a placebo or a combination of *Lactobacillus rhamnosus* GG and LC705, *Bifidobacterium breve* Bb99, and *Propionibacterium freudenreichii* ssp. *shermanii* for four weeks prior to delivery. Their infants were given the same formula together with prebiotics, or a placebo for 6 months after birth. During the infants' six-month treatment period, antibiotics were prescribed less often among the probiotic group by 23%. In addition, respiratory infections occurred less frequently among the probiotic group through the two-year follow-up period (even after treatment had stopped) compared to the placebo group (an average of 3.7 infections versus 4.2 infections).

Finnish scientists (Kirjavainen *et al.* 2002) gave 21 infants with early onset atopic eczema a placebo or *Bifidobacterium lactis* Bb-12. Serum IgE concentration correlated directly to *Escherichia coli* and bacteroides counts, indicating the association between these bacteria with atopic sensitization. The probiotic group had a decrease in the numbers of *Escherichia coli* and bacteroides.

Researchers from Italy's University G. D'Annunzio (Di Marzio *et al.* 2003) applied sonicated *Streptococcus thermophilus* cream to the forearms of 11 patients with atopic dermatitis for two weeks. This led to a significant increase of skin ceramide levels, and a significant improvement of their clinical signs and symptoms—including erythema, scaling and pruritus.

Japanese researchers (Odamaki *et al.* 2007) gave yogurt with *Bifidobacterium longum* BB536 or plain yogurt to 40 patients with Japanese cedar pollinosis for 14 weeks. *Bacteroides fragilis* significantly changed with pollen dispersion. The ratio of *B. fragilis* to bifidobacteria also increased significantly during pollen season among the placebo group but not in the *B. longum* group. Peripheral blood mononuclear cells from the patients indicated that *B. fragilis* microorganisms induced significantly more Th2 cell cytokines such as interleukin-6, and fewer Th1 cell cytokines such as IL-12 and interferon. The researchers concluded that, *"These re-*

sults suggest a relationship between fluctuation in intestinal microbiota and pollinosis allergy. Furthermore, intake of BB536 yogurt appears to exert positive influences on the formation of antiallergic microbiota."

Scientists from the Department of Oral Microbiology at Japan's Asahi University School of Dentistry (Ogawa *et al.* 2006) studied skin allergic symptoms and blood chemistry of healthy human volunteers during the cedar pollen season in Japan. After supplementation with *Lactobacillus casei*, activity of cedar pollen-specific IgE, thymus, chemokines, eosinophils, and interferon-gamma levels all decreased among the probiotic group.

Researchers from the School of Medicine and Health Sciences in Wellington, New Zealand (Sistek *et al.* 2006) determined in a study of *Lactobacillus rhamnosus* and *Bifidobacteria lactis* on 59 children with established atopic dermatitis that food-sensitized children responded significantly better to probiotics than did other atopic dermatitis children.

French scientists (Passeron *et al.* 2006) found that atopic dermatitis children improved significantly after three months of *Lactobacillus rhamnosus* treatment, based on SCORAD levels of 39.1 before and 20.7 after probiotic supplementation.

Scientists from Finland's National Public Health Institute (Piirainen *et al.* 2008) gave a placebo or *Lactobacillus rhamnosus* GG to 38 patients with atopic eczema for 5.5 months—starting 2.5 months before birch pollen season. Saliva and serum samples taken before and after indicated that allergen-specific IgA levels increased significantly among the probiotic group versus the placebo group (using the enzyme-linked immunosorbent assay (ELISA)). Allergen-specific IgE levels correlated positively with stimulated IgA and IgG in saliva, while they correlated negatively in the placebo group. The researchers concluded that the research showed that *L. rhamnosus* GG displayed *"immunostimulating effects on oral mucosa seen as increased allergen specific IgA levels in saliva."*

Children with cow's milk allergy and IgE-associated dermatitis were given a placebo or *Lactobacillus rhamnosus* GG and a combination of four other probiotic bacteria (Pohjavuori *et al.* 2004). The IFN-gamma by PBMCs at the beginning of supplementation was significantly lower among cow's milk allergy infants. However, cow's milk allergy infants receiving *L. rhamnosus* GG had significantly increased levels of IFN-gamma, showing increased tolerance.

The British medical publication *Lancet* published a study (Kalliomäki *et al.* 2003) where 107 children with a high risk of atopic eczema were given either a placebo or *Lactobacillus rhamnosus* GG during their first two years of life. Fourteen of 53 children receiving the probiotic developed atopic eczema, while 25 of 54 of the children receiving the placebo contracted atopic eczema by the end of the study.

In a study from the University of Western Australia School of Pediatrics (Taylor *et al.* 2006), 178 children born of mothers with allergies were given either *Lactobacillus acidophilus* or a placebo for the first six months of life. Those given the probiotics showed reduced levels of IL-5 and TGF-beta in response to polyclonal stimulation (typical for allergic responses), and significantly lower IL-10 responses to vaccines compared to the placebo group. This illustrated that the probiotics increased allergen resistance.

Researchers from the Department of Otolaryngology and Sensory Organ Surgery at Osaka University School of Medicine in Japan (Tamura *et al.* 2007) studied allergic response in chronic rhinitis patients. For eight weeks, patients were given either a placebo or *Lactobacillus casei* strain Shirota. Those with moderate-to-severe nasal symptom scores at the beginning of the study who were given probiotics experienced significantly reduced nasal symptoms.

Intestinal Permeability

Earlier we introduced the possible connection between allergies and intestinal permeability. In recent years, research on intestinal drug absorption by the pharmaceutical industry confirmed that the lining of the small intestine is subject to alteration, dramatically affecting absorption and permeability. As this research has progressed, it has become apparent that nutrient absorption can be significantly altered by changes in the intestinal wall. Worse, increased intestinal permeability syndrome (IIPS) has been implicated in many allergic and arthritic conditions.

This link is related to the fact that permeability allows macromolecules—larger peptides, toxins and even invading microorganisms—into the bloodstream. Once these foreigners arrive in the bloodstream, the immune system may activate a variety of inflammatory responses as a defense measure. For example, the invasion of pathogenic microorganisms through the intestinal wall can result in bacterial translocation throughout the body—stimulating inflammatory responses (Baik 2004; Yasuda *et al.* 2006). Illustrating this mechanism, *Blastocystis hominis*—pathogenic bacteria typically found in the intestines—have been found within synovial (joint) membranes of arthritic patients (Kruger *et al.* 1994).

The intestinal brush barrier is a complex mucosal layer of enzymes, probiotics and ionic fluid. It forms a protective surface medium over the intestinal epithelium. It also provides an active nutrient transport mechanism. This mucosal layer is stabilized by the grooves of the intestinal microvilli. It contains glycoproteins and other ionic transporters, which attach to nutrient molecules, carrying them across intestinal membranes. This transport medium requires a delicately pH-balanced mix of ionic chemistry able to facilitate this transport of amino acids, minerals, vitamins, glucose and fatty acids. The mucosal layer is policed by billions of probiotic colonies, which help process incoming food molecules, excrete various nutrients, and control pathogens. In a healthy mucosal environment, probiotics will also produce several B vitamins and potent antibiotics (DeWill and Kudsk 1999).

This probiotic-rich mucosal brush barrier creates the boundary between intestinal contents and our bloodstream. Should the mucosal layer chemistry become altered, its protective and ionic transport mechanisms become weakened, allowing toxic or larger molecules to be presented to the microvilli junctions. This contact can irritate the microvilli, causing a subsequent inflammatory response. This is now considered a contributing cause of various intestinal disorders such as IBS and Crohn's disease.

Intestinal permeability and the reduction of probiotic colonies among the intestinal wall are caused by a number of factors. Alcohol is one of the most irritating substances to the intestinal lining and the health of our probiotic colonies (Ferrier *et al.* 2006; Bongaerts and Severijnen 2005). In addition, many pharmaceutical drugs, notably NSAIDs, have been identified as damaging to the mucosal chemistry and probiotic populations. Foods with high arachidonic fatty acid capability (such as trans-fats and animal meats); low-fiber, high-glucose foods; and high nitrite-forming foods have also been observed as compromising the intestinal lining. Toxic substances such as plasticizers, pesticides, herbicides, chlorinated water and food dyes also reduce the integrity of these tissues and flora. In general, substances that increase PGE-2 response—inflammation—tend to increase permeability (Martin-Venegas *et al.* 2006).

In addition, the overuse of antibiotics causes a die-off of resident probiotic colonies. When intestinal probiotic colonies are decreased, pathogenic bacteria and yeasts can outgrow probiotic colonies near the intestinal lining. Pathogenic bacteria growth invades the brush barrier, introducing an influx of endotoxins (the waste matter of these microorganisms) into the bloodstream. This is also sometimes accompanied by the pathogenic microorganisms getting in themselves.

Inflammatory responses resulting from IIPS has been linked with sinusitis, allergies, psoriasis, asthma, arthritis and other inflammatory disorders. Overgrowth of *Candida albicans,* a typical fungal inhabitant of the digestive system at controlled populations, has also been attributed to IIPS. Systemic Candida infections have a route of translocation via IIPS. The research has also supported a link between intestinal permeability and liver damage (Bode and Bode 2003).

In a study by scientists from China's Qilu Hospital and Shandong University (Zeng *et al.* 2008), 30 irritable bowel syndrome patients with intestinal wall permeability were given either a placebo or a fermented milk beverage with *Streptococcus thermophilus, Lactobacillus bulgaricus, Lactobacillus acidophilus* and *Bifidobacterium longum.* After four weeks, intestinal permeability reduced significantly among the probiotic group.

Researchers from Greece's Alexandra Regional General Hospital (Stratiki *et al.* 2007) gave 41 preterm infants of 27-36 weeks gestation a formula supplemented with *Bifidobacterium lactis* or a placebo. After 7 days, bifidobacteria counts were significantly higher, head growth was greater, and the lactulose/mannitol ratio (a marker for intestinal permeability) was significantly lower after 30 days in the probiotic group as compared to the placebo group. The researchers concluded that, *"bifidobacteria supplemented infant formula decreases intestinal permeability of preterm infants and leads to increased head growth."*

Granada medical researchers (Lara-Villoslada *et al.* 2007) gave *Lactobacillus coryniformis* CECT5711 and *Lactobacillus gasseri* CECT5714 or a placebo to 30 healthy children after having received conventional yogurt containing *Lactobacillus bulgaricus* and *Streptococcus thermophilus* for three weeks. The supplemented yogurt significantly inhibited *Salmonella cholerasuis* adhesion to intestinal mucins compared to before probiotic supplementation. The probiotic supplementation also increased IgA concentration in feces and saliva from the oral cavity.

German scientists (Rosenfeldt *et al.* 2004) gave *Lactobacillus rhamnosus* 19070-2 and *L. reuteri* DSM 12246 or a placebo to 41 children. After six weeks of treatment, the frequency of GI symptoms were significantly lower (10% versus 39%) among the probiotic group as compared to the placebo group. In addition, the lactulose-to-mannitol ratio was lower in the probiotic group, indicating to the researchers that, *"probiotic supplementation may stabilize the intestinal barrier function and decrease gastrointestinal symptoms in children with atopic dermatitis."*

Researchers from the People's Hospital and the Jiao Tong University in Shangha (Qin *et al.* 2008) gave *Lactobacillus plantarum* or placebo to 76 patients with acute pancreatitis. Intestinal permeability was determined using the lactulose/rhamnose ratio. Incidences of organ failure, septic complications and death were also monitored. After 7 days of treatment, microbial infections averaged 38.9% in the probiotic group and 73.7% in the placebo group. 30.6% of the probiotic group colonized potentially pathogenic organisms, as compared to 50% of patients in the control group. The probiotic group also had significantly better clinical outcomes compared to the control group. The researchers concluded that *Lactobacillus plantarum "can attenuate disease severity, improve the intestinal permeability and clinical outcomes."*

Ulcers

Just a couple of decades ago, medical scientists and physicians were certain that ulcers were caused by too much acid in the stomach and the eating of spicy foods. This assumption has been debunked over the past two decades as researchers have confirmed that at least 80% of all ulcers are associated with *Helicobacter pylori* infections.

While acidic foods and gastrin produced by the stomach wall are also implicated with symptoms of heartburn and acid reflux, we know that a healthy stomach has a functional barrier that should prevent these normal food and gastric substances from harming the cells of the stomach wall. This barrier is called the mucosal membrane. This stomach's mucosal membrane contains a number of mucopolysaccharides and phospholipids that, together with secretions from intestinal and oral probiotics, protect the stomach cells from acids, toxins and bacteria invasions.

As doctors and researchers work to eradicate *H. pylori,* which infects billions of people worldwide, they are finding that *H. pylori* is becoming increasingly resistant to many of the antibiotics used in prescriptive treatment. Research from Poland's Center of Gastrology (Ziemniak 2006) investigated antibiotic use on *Helicobacter pylori* infections: 641 *H. pylori* patients were given various antibiotics typically applied to *H. pylori*. The results indicated that *H. pylori* had developed a 22% resistance to clarithromycin and 47% resistance to metronidazole. Worse, a 66% secondary resistance to clarithromycin and metronidazole was found, indicating *H. pylori's* increasing resistance to antibiotics.

H. pylori bacteria do not always cause ulcers. In fact, only a small percentage of *H. pylori* infections actually become ulcerative. Meanwhile, there is some evidence that *H. pylori*—like *E. coli* and *Candida albicans*—may be a normal resident in a healthy intestinal tract, assuming it is properly balanced and managed by strong legions of probiotics.

Here are some research data that confirms the ability probiotics have in controlling and managing *H. pylori* overgrowths. Here we will also see probiotics' ability to arrest ulcerative colitis and even mouth ulcers:

Researchers from the Academic Hospital at Vrije University in The Netherlands (Cats *et al.* 2003) gave either a placebo or *Lactobacillus casei* Shirota to 14 *H. pylori*-infected patients for three weeks. Six additional *H. pylori*-infected subjects were used as controls. The researchers determined that *L. casei* significantly inhibits *H. pylori* growth. This effect was more pronounced for *L. casei* grown in milk solution than in the DeMan-Rogosa-Sharpe medium (a probiotic broth developed by researchers in 1960).

Mexican hospital researchers (Sahagún-Flores *et al.* 2007) gave 64 *Helicobacter pylori*-infected patients antibiotic treatment with or without *Lactobacillus casei* Shirota. *Lactobacillus casei* Shirota plus antibiotic treatment was 94% effective and antibiotic treatment alone was 76% effective.

Researchers from the Department of Internal Medicine and Gastroenterology at Italy's University of Bologna (Gionchetti *et al.* 2000) gave 40 ulcerative colitis patients either a placebo or a combination of four strains of lactobacilli, three strains of bifidobacteria, and one strain of *Streptococcus salivarius* subsp. *thermo-*

philus for nine months. The patients were tested monthly. Three patients (15%) in the probiotic group suffered relapses within the nine months, versus 20 (100%) in the placebo group.

Italian scientists from the University of Bologna (Venturi *et al.* 1999) also gave 20 patients with ulcerative colitis a combination of three bifidobacteria strains, four lactobacilli strains and *Streptococcus salivarius* subsp. *thermophilus* for 12 months. Fecal samples were obtained at the beginning, after 10 days, 20 days, 40 days, 60 days, 75 days, 90 days, 12 months and 15 days after the (12 months) end of the treatment period. Fifteen of the 20 treated patients achieved and maintained remission from ulcerative colitis during the study period.

British researchers from the University of Dundee and Ninewells Hospital Medical School (Furrie *et al.* 2005) gave 18 patients with active ulcerative colitis either *B. longum* or a placebo for one month. Clinical examination and rectal biopsies indicated that sigmoidoscopy scores were reduced in the probiotic group. In addition, mRNA levels for human beta defensins 2, 3, and 4 (higher in active ulcerative colitis) were significantly reduced among the probiotic group. Inflammatory cytokines tumor necrosis factor alpha and interleukin-1alpha were also significantly lower in the probiotic group. Biopsies showed reduced inflammation and the regeneration of epithelial tissue within the intestines among the probiotic group.

Scientists from Italy's Raffaele University Hospital (Guslandi *et al.* 2003) gave *Saccharomyces boulardii* or placebo to 25 patients with ulcerative colitis unsuitable for steroid therapy, for 4 weeks. Of the 24 patients completing the study, 17 attained clinical remission, which was confirmed endoscopically.

Researchers from Switzerland's University Hospital in Lausanne (Felley *et al.* 2001) gave fifty-three patients with ulcerative *H. pylori* infection milk with *L. johnsonii* or placebo for three weeks. Those given the probiotic drink had a significant *H. pylori* density decrease, reduced inflammation and less gastritis activity from *H. pylori*.

Lactobacillus reuteri ATCC 55730 or a placebo was given to 40 *H. pylori*-infected patients for 4 weeks by researchers from Italy's Università degli Studi di Bari (Francavilla *et al.* 2008). *L. reuteri* effectively suppressed *H. pylori* infection, decreased gastrointestinal pain, and reduced other dyspeptic symptoms.

Scientists from the Department of Internal Medicine at the Catholic University of Rome (Canducci *et al.* 2000) tested 120 patients with ulcerative *H. pylori* infections. Sixty patients received a combination of antibiotics rabeprazole, clarithromycin and amoxicillin. The other sixty patients received the same therapy together with a freeze-dried, inactivated culture of *Lactobacillus acidophilus*. The probiotic group had an 88% eradication of *H. pylori* while the antibiotic-only group had a 72% eradication of *H. pylori*.

Scientists from the University of Chile (Gotteland *et al.* 2005) gave 182 children with *H. pylori* infections placebo, antibiotics or probiotics. *H. pylori* were completely eradicated in 12% of those who took *Saccharomyces boulardii*, and in 6.5% of those given *L. acidophilus*. The placebo group had no *H. pylori* eradication.

Researchers from Japan's Kyorin University School of Medicine (Imase *et al.* 2007) gave *Lactobacillus reuteri* strain SD2112 in tablets or a placebo to 33 *H. pylori*-infected patients. After 4 and 8 weeks, *L. reuteri* significantly decreased and suppressed *H. pylori* in the probiotic group.

In a study of 347 patients with active *H. pylori* infections (ulcerous), half the group was given antibiotics and the other half was given antibiotics with yogurt (*Lactobacillus acidophilus* HY2177, *Lactobacillus casei* HY2743, *Bifidobacterium longum* HY8001, and *Streptococcus thermophilus* B-1). The yogurt plus antibiotics group had significantly more eradication of the *H. pylori* bacteria, and significantly less side effects than the antibiotics group (Kim, *et al.* 2008).

Lactobacillus brevis (CD2) or placebo was given to 22 *H. pylori*-positive dyspeptic patients for three weeks before a colonoscopy by Italian medical researchers (Linsalata *et al.* 2004). A reduction in the UBT delta values and subsequent bacterial load ensued. *L. brevis* CD2 stimulated a decrease in gastric ornithine decarboxylase activity and polyamine. The researchers concluded: *"Our data support the hypothesis that L. brevis CD2 treatment decreases H. pylori colonization, thus reducing polyamine biosynthesis."*

Thirty *H. pylori*-infected patients were given either probiotics *Lactobacillus acidophilus* and *Bifidobacterium bifidum* or placebo for one and two weeks following antibiotic treatment by British researchers (Madden *et al.* 2005). Those taking the probiotics had a recovery of normal intestinal microflora, damaged during antibiotic treatment. The researchers also observed that those taking the probiotics throughout the two weeks showed more normal and stable microflora than did those groups taking the probiotics for only one out of the two weeks.

Researchers at the Nippon Medical School in Tokyo (Fujimori *et al.* 2009) gave 120 outpatients with ulcerative colitis either a placebo; *Bifidobacterium longum;* psyllium (a prebiotic); or a combination of *B. longum* and psyllium (synbiotics) for four weeks. C-reactive protein (pro-inflammatory) decreased significantly only with the synbiotic group, from 0.59 to 0.14 mg/dL. In addition, the synbiotic therapy experienced significantly better scores on symptom and quality-of-life assessment.

Scientists from the Department of Medicine at Lausanne, Switzerland's University Hospital (Michetti *et al.* 1999) tested 20 human adults with ulcerative *H. pylori* infection with *L. acidophilus johnsonii*. The probiotic was taken with the antibiotic omeprazole in half the group and alone (with placebo) in the other group. The patients were tested at the start, after two weeks of treatment, and four weeks after treatment. Both groups showed significantly reduced *H. pylori* levels during and just following treatment. However, the probiotic-only group tested better than the antibiotic group during the fourth week after the treatment completion.

Medical scientists from the Kaohsiung Municipal United Hospital in Taiwan (Wang *et al.* 2004) studied 59 volunteer patients infected with *H. pylori*. They were given either probiotics (*Lactobacillus* and *Bifidobacterium* strains) or placebo after meals for six weeks. After the six-week treatment period, the probiotic group *"effectively suppressed H. pylori,"* according to the researchers.

In the Polish study mentioned earlier (Ziemniak 2006), 641 *H. pylori* patients were given either antibiotics alone or probiotics with antibiotics. The two antibiotic-only treatment groups had 71% and 86% eradication of *H. pylori,* while the antibiotic-probiotic treatment group had 94% eradication.

Researchers from the Cerrahpasa Medical Faculty at Istanbul University (Tasli *et al.* 2006) gave 25 patients with Behçet's syndrome (chronic mouth ulcers) six *Lactobacillus brevis* CD2 lozenges per day at intervals of 2-3 hours. After one and two weeks, the number of ulcers significantly decreased.

Vaginosis and Vaginitis

A healthy vagina is lined with probiotic bacteria just as the mouth is. These bacteria protect the woman's internal tissues and organs from being overwhelmed by pathogenic bacteria, yeasts and other pathogens. Without a balance of probiotic bacteria, overgrowths can take place easily. Normal colonies within a healthy vagina include lactobacilli, *Gardenella vaginalis, Candida albicans* and other microorganisms—all existing in balance.

Vaginosis is the alteration of the normal microbiological ecology. Vaginitis is an overgrowth of pathogenic bacteria, and their resulting infection. Two common infective microorganisms within the vagina are *Candida albicans* and *Trichomonas vaginalis.* The use of antibiotics, antiseptics and chemical toxins can stress probiotic populations, allowing further imbalances and overgrowths to take place.

Vaginitis can easily lead to urinary tract infections as pathogenic bacteria colonies expand. Vagina bacterial infection is often symptomized by stinging sensations and a fishy odor from the vagina. As we'll discuss later and as indicated in the research, internal supplementation (through the mouth) and external application (into the vagina) both have been shown to help replenish the probiotic populations within the vagina.

Estrogen production can also be a factor. Researchers from Israel's HaEmek Medical Center (Colodner *et al.* 2003) determined from research that, *"The lack of lactobacilli in the vagina of postmenopausal women due to estrogen deficiency plays an important role in the development of bacteriuria."*

Researchers from the School of Medicine at Italy's Università degli Studi di Siena (Delia *et al.* 2006) treated 60 healthy women with vaginosis with either a vaginal suppository containing *Lactobacillus acidophilus* or a suppository containing *Lactobacillus acidophilus* and *Lactobacillus paracasei* F19. At the end of three months of treatment—and again three months afterward—both groups showed significant improvement in vaginosis, a significant reduction in vaginal pH, and significant decrease in vagina odor.

In a study from the University of Milan (Drago *et al.* 2007), forty women with vaginosis took a douche with *Lactobacillus acidophilus* for six days. After treatment, only 7.5% of the women still had the vaginosis. The odor typical in vaginosis discontinued in all the women, and the pH went to normal levels of 4.5 in 34 of the 40 women.

Scientists from the University of Western Ontario (Reid *et al.* 2001) gave 42 women oral encapsulated *Lactobacillus rhamnosus* GR-1 plus *Lactobacillus fermentum* RC-14 probiotics, or *L. rhamno-*

sus GG orally for 28 days. Vaginal flora—normal in only 40% of the cases—resolved to healthy flora in 90% of the women in the GR-1 group, and the 7 of 11 women with bacterial vaginosis at the beginning of the study were resolved within a month. *L. rhamnosus* GG did not have an effect.

In a similar study (Reid *et al.* 2003), 64 women were given placebo or *Lactobacillus rhamnosus* GR-1 and *Lactobacillus fermentum* RC-14 daily for 60 days. The treatment resulted in the restoration from bacterial vaginosis microflora to normal lactobacilli-colonized microflora in 37% of the women treated with the probiotic, versus only 13% among the placebo group.

Researchers from Israel's Central Emek Hospital (Shalev *et al.* 1996) gave 46 bacterial vaginosis patients either yogurt with live *L acidophilus* or a placebo for several months. The probiotic group had significantly less vaginosis than the control group.

Researchers from Sweden's Uppsala University Hospital (Hallén *et al.* 1992) gave 60 women infected with bacterial vaginosis either a placebo or *Lactobacillus acidophilus*. At the end of the study, 16 of the 28 women treated with lactobacilli had normal vaginal wet smear results while no improvement occurred among the 29 women treated with the placebo. Infective vagina bacteroides were eliminated from 12 of 16 women in the probiotic group.

Italian scientists (Cianci *et al.* 2008) investigated the use of *Lactobacillus rhamnosus* GR-1 and *Lactobacillus reuteri* for the treatment and prevention of vaginosis and bacterial vaginitis. Fifty women with diagnosed bacterial vaginosis and vaginitis took either a placebo or an oral combination of *Lactobacillus rhamnosus* GR-1 and *Lactobacillus reuteri* RC-14 following antibiotic therapy. The researchers found that 92% of the patients significantly benefited from the probiotic treatment.

Scientists from Brazil's Universidade de Sao Paulo (Martinez *et al.* 2009) gave 64 women with bacterial vaginosis tinidazole with placebo or with a combination of oral *Lactobacillus rhamnosus* GR-1 and *Lactobacillus reuteri* RC-14 daily for four weeks. The probiotic group experienced a cure rate of 87%, while the placebo group experienced a 50% cure rate. Normal vagina flora resumed in 75% of the probiotic group and in only 34% of the placebo group. This research team (2009) found similar results in another study on 55 women with vulvovaginal candidiasis.

Researchers from the Department of Obstetrics and Fetomaternal Medicine at Austria's Medical University of Vienna (Petricevic and Witt 2008) tested 190 women with bacterial vaginosis. They were given either placebo or topical plus oral *Lactobacillus rhamnosus* after antibiotic treatment for 7 days. Sixty-nine of 83 (or 83%) in the probiotic group significantly improved, versus 31 of the 88 women (35%) in the placebo group.

Another study done by researchers from the Medical University of Vienna (Petricevic *et al.* 2008) gave *Lactobacillus rhamnosus* GR-1 and *Lactobacillus reuteri* RC-14 or placebo to 72 postmenopausal women with vaginosis for seven days. Both the placebo group and the probiotic group had received antibiotic treatment for seven days prior. Four weeks after treatment concluded, 60% (21 of 35) of the probiotic group demonstrated a significant improvement, while only 6 of the 37 non-probiotic subjects (16%) showed the same level of improvement.

Candida Infections

Candida albicans is a normal inhabitant of the intestinal tract, the upper respiratory tract, and several other locations throughout the body. Complications arise when *Candida* populations have been allowed to grow beyond their normal levels. Reduced probiotic populations allow these fungi to grow beyond their functional levels, infecting the intestines, vagina and many other parts of the body. The consumption of probiotics can help return *Candida* back to its normal population levels, as probiotics manage and control their colonies by secreting chemicals that limit their growth.

Researchers from Long Island Jewish Medical Center's Division of Infectious Diseases (Hilton, *et al.* 1992) studied thirty-three patients with vulvovaginal candida infections. Infection rates decreased by a third among patients consuming an eight-ounce yogurt (orally) with *Lactobacillus acidophilus* for six months. The average infection rate was 2.54 in the control group versus 0.38 in the yogurt group, while *Candida* spp. colonization rates were 3.23 in the control group versus only 0.84 in the yogurt group— throughout the six-month testing period.

Baby Colic

Colic is the incessant crying of a baby, often resulting in dramatic oxygen reduction and other complications. Conventional medicine is still mystified by colic. There are a number of theories as to its cause. Some believe it has more to do with nutrition or perhaps their environment. Others believe that bacterial infection is the main cause. Studies with probiotics give us another perspective on this mystery.

Researchers at Johns Hopkins University School of Medicine (Saavedra *et al.* 2004) gave a *Bifidobacterium lactis* and *Streptococcus thermophilus* combination or a placebo to 118 infants (average age 2.9 months) for 210 days. The probiotic group had a significantly lower frequency of colic and irritability, and a lower need (frequency) for antibiotics than did the placebo group.

Italian researchers from the University of Bari Policlinico (Indrio *et al.* 2008) gave 30 preterm newborns either a placebo or *Lactobacillus reuteri* ATCC 55730 for 30 days. Newborns fed with probiotics had a significant reduction in regurgitation and mean daily crying time.

Researchers from Italy's Regina Margherita Children's Hospital (Savino *et al.* 2007) gave either simethicone (colic medication) or *Lactobacillus reuteri* to 90 children with infantile colic. After 28 days, 39 patients (95%) responded positively among the probiotic group, while only three patients (7%) responded positively among the simethicone group. Colicky symptoms among breastfed infants in the *L. reuteri* group improved within 1 week of treatment.

Ear Infections

Most of us would laugh at the prospect that probiotics would help or prevent ear infections. Think again.

Scientists from Sweden's University of Gothenburg (Skovbjerg *et al.* 2009) studied the effect of probiotic treatment on secretory otitis media—an ear infection with fluid in the middle ear cavity. Sixty children suffering from chronic secretory otitis media who were scheduled for tympanostomy tube insertion were given a nasal spray of placebo, *Streptococcus sanguinis* or *Lactobacillus rhamnosus* for 10 days prior to surgery. *"Complete or significant clinical recovery"* occurred in 7 of 19 patients treated with *S. sanguinis;* in 3 of 18 patients treated with *L. rhamnosus;* and only in 1 of 17 of the placebo patients.

Researchers from Finland's University of Turku (Rautava *et al.* 2009) gave infant formula supplemented with either a placebo or *Lactobacillus rhamnosus GG* and *Bifidobacterium lactis Bb-12* from two months of age to 12 months. Ear infection rates among the probiotic group were 22%, while 50% of the placebo infants experienced ear infections through seven months.

Anorexia Nervosa

Modern medicine classifies anorexia nervosa as a psychological disorder. Most people who have anorexia nervosa, however, will likely say otherwise. While many who have anorexia nervosa are characterized by an excessive compulsion to lose weight or appear attractive to others, there are also biological components to the disease. A person with anorexia has also lost the physical desire to eat. A person with anorexia nervosa also has the same lack of physical desire, but this will be accompanied by anxiety about their weight or appearance. In both cases, other things are more important than eating. This, however, has a biological component because a proper appetite has not been developed in either case. In a healthy person, there may also be anxiety about appearance, but there will still be hunger.

Anxiety stresses more than just our minds. When we are anxious, our adrenal glands begin to produce stress chemicals such as adrenaline. This is accompanied by a mechanism that shuts down our appetite. Our vagus nerve is stimulated in a way that decreases our stomach's output of mucopolysaccharides and gastrin. Our salivary glands slow down their production of enzymes such as amylase. Our body's appetite for food is put aside to make way for the stressor of the moment. This is mirrored by a stimulated immune system, which further shuts down the body's ability to produce the right chemistry for digestion and appetite.

This stress, and the resulting chemistry produced by it, deters the growth of our probiotics in our mouth and stomach. In other words, stress directly reduces probiotic populations. With this reduction comes a reduced inclination to eat and digest foods. It is a vicious cycle, in which our innocent probiotic friends become victims of our mind's anxieties, and our body's physical response to stress.

Illustrating this connection, scientists from Spain (Nova *et al.* 2006) gave yogurt with *L. bulgaricus* and *S. thermophilus* or placebo to 16 anorexia nervosa (AN) adolescent patients and 15 healthy adolescents for ten weeks. Blood lymphocyte levels were measured, revealing that the probiotics stimulated increased CD8+ cytokine subset and IFN-gamma production, which help modify the body's nutritional response to stress. The researchers concluded: *"The findings suggest that the inclusion of yogurt in the refeeding therapy of AN patients may exert positive effects on the immunological markers related to the nutritional status of these pa-*

tients, such as the CD4+/CD8+ ratio and the production of IFN-gamma by lymphocytes."

Keratoconjunctivitis

Keratoconjunctivitis is an inflammation of the conjunctiva of the eyes. As in most forms of inflammation, this can be due to toxins, infection, stress or lacrimal dryness (lacrimal gland malfunction). Pathogenic endotoxins and bacteria are often the cause of these issues. The immune system launches an inflammatory attack to resolve the situation and clear out the toxins and/or pathogens. This is where probiotics come in. There is some evidence that probiotics might also be dwelling within the lacrimal fluids of eye. This is supported by research showing the improvement of keratoconjunctivitis with probiotics:

Medical researchers from the University of Rome (Iovieno *et al.* 2008) gave seven patients with vernal keratoconjunctivitis eye drops with *Lactobacillus acidophilus* for four weeks. After treatment, 6 of 7 showed significant improvement of clinical symptoms after two weeks of treatment. These symptoms included itching, photophobia and burning. In addition, clinical signs—such as conjunctiva hyperemia, chemosis, secretion, Trantas dots and superficial punctuate keratitis—all showed significant improvement among the patients after the four weeks of probiotic treatment.

Viral Infections

The stimulation of the immune system by probiotics has also been observed among some of the most pervasive viral infections known to humankind. These include rhinovirus (colds), influenza virus (flu), rotavirus (intestinal infection) and even herpes viruses.

Viral influenza is now a critical issue among medical experts. With the advent of the H1N1 swine flu virus and other seasonal flu infections, influenza threatens millions of people. While some have quoted statistics that from 25,000 to 35,000 people die each year of influenza, upon closer examination, well over 90% of those actually are immunosuppressed persons who die of pneumonia. Whether the flu or pneumonia is the official cause of death, the reason for these deaths is an overburdened and weakened immune system, not necessarily the flu or pneumonia itself.

Furthermore, despite valiant efforts by so many researchers over many decades, the "cure for the common cold" still eludes modern medicine. For most immune systems, this virus is not such a problem, because we typically can get over a cold within a few days. However, for those who are immunosuppressed, a simple cold can easily turn into pneumonia and other respiratory infections. In fact, many elderly people die from infections that began with a simple cold or the flu as mentioned above.

We are now faced with more risk of virulent influenza and other infectious outbreaks due to transcontinental flights and world travelers. Can probiotics help stave off viral infections? More importantly, can probiotics fight dangerous influenza viruses like H1N1? The answer lies in the ability of probiotics to specifically stimulate the immune system and attack foreign microorganisms.

German scientists (de Vrese *et al.* 2005) gave a placebo or *Lactobacillus gasseri*, *Bifidobacterium longum* and *Bifidobacterium bifidum* to 479 healthy adult volunteers for three months. Total symptom score, duration of cold illness, and fever duration were significantly lower among the probiotic group—shortening common cold episodes by about 2 days—with a score of 79.3 versus 102.5 points. The probiotic group had significantly higher levels of cytotoxic T suppressor cells (CD8+) and higher activity among T helper cells (CD4+), along with reduced severity of symptoms.

In a study mentioned earlier, Finnish medical researchers from the University of Turku (Rautava *et al.* 2009) gave infants younger than two months of age either formula supplemented with *Lactobacillus rhamnosus* GG and *Bifidobacterium lactis* Bb-12 or formula with a placebo daily until they were 12 months of age. Incidence of respiratory infections was 28% among the probiotic infants and 55% among the placebo group.

In research that began in the late 1950s, Dr. Don Weekes clinically administered a combination of *L. acidophilus* and *L. bulgaricus* to 180 patients with ulcers and/or herpes viral infections. After average treatment times of three days with four-times daily doses, 61 of 64 patients with herpes simplex labialis, 77 of 97 patients with mouth ulcers (aphthous stomatitis), 6 of 13 patients with dendrites ulcers, and 6 of 6 patients with genital herpes were either *"cured"* or *"much improved"* from the probiotic treatments (Trenev 1998; Weekes 1983; Weekes 1958).

Bulgarian researchers have also confirmed herpes simplex inhibition from species of lactobacilli (Dimitonova *et al.* 2007).

One hundred children from a slum of New Delhi between two and five years old were given either a probiotic curd with *Lactobacillus acidophilus* or a placebo for six months. The probiotic group had more growth, and had fewer incidences of colds, flu, diarrhea and fever than the placebo group (Saran *et al.* 2002).

Scientists from Finland's University of Tampere (Isolauri *et al.* 1995) studied the administration of *Lactobacillus casei* GG with oral rotavirus vaccines given to 2-5-month-old infants. Infants receiving the probiotic displayed an increased level of rotavirus-specific IgM secreting cells. The researchers concluded that, *"these findings suggest that LGG has an immunostimulating effect on oral rotavirus vaccination."*

Scientists from Taiwan's Buddhist Tzu Chi General Hospital (Lin *et al.* 2009) gave 1,062 children under the age of five a placebo or *L. rhamnosus.* The children given the probiotic had significantly lower rates of bacterial, viral and respiratory infections, along with increased T-cell activity.

Swedish researchers (Tubelius *et al.* 2005) gave 262 healthy employees at Sweden's TetraPak company either *L. reuteri* or placebo for 80 days. During the study, the placebo group's sick leave reporting was 26.4% compared to 10.6% among the *L. reuteri* group. The sick-day frequency was 0.9% among the placebo group and 0.4% among the *L. reuteri* group. Among 53 shift-workers, 33% in the placebo group reported being sick during the study period as compared to none in the *L. reuteri* group.

Lactobacillus casei DN-114001 was given to 360 elderly people for 3 weeks by Italian researchers (Turchet *et al.* 2003). The probiotic group suffered a 20% shorter duration of winter illnesses compared to the placebo group.

Scientists from Italy's University of Milan (Pregliasco *et al.* 2008) gave placebo or several combinations of *Lactobacillus plantarum*, *Lactobacillus rhamnosus*, and *Bifidobacterium lactis* together with prebiotics to healthy volunteers over three winter seasons (2003-2007). Acute respiratory infection episodes and upper respiratory tract infections were significantly lower among the probiotic groups. Severity of all illness episodes decreased significantly among probiotic groups, ranging from .73 days less to 1.12 days less in average duration compared to the placebo groups. The duration of upper respiratory infections ranged from 1.51 days less to 2.07 days less than the placebo groups. The probiotic groups also had an average of 1.25 to 1.4 days less flu illnesses than the placebo groups. There was also significantly fewer cold illnesses among the probiotics groups compared to the placebo groups.

Halitosis (Bad Breath) and Dry Mouth

Pathogenic oral bacteria produce volatile sulfur compounds like hydrogen sulfide. These compounds cause sour breath. Periodontal disease-causing bacteria such as *Streptococcus mutans, Streptococcus pyogenes, Porphyromonas gingivalis, Veillonella* sp., *Actinomyces* sp., and *Prevotella* sp. have been pinpointed as producing halitosis among humans (Washio *et al.* 2005). These sour colonies indicate a reduction of probiotic species such as *Lactobacillus salivarius* that control sulfur-producing bacteria.

Halitosis bacteria often accumulate at the back of the tongue, in the pharynx and around the gums. They are difficult to remove. Alcohol and chlorhexidine mouthwashes are typical prescriptions. These do not completely remove the bacteria, but merely temporarily reduce colonies. Once the mouthwash subsides, the colonies simply regrow in the absence of their competitors, oral probiotics.

Several studies have illustrated supplementing *Streptococcus salivarius* or *Lactobacillus reuteri* can change the relative strength and activities of halitosis bacteria.

New Zealand's University of Otago researchers (Burton *et al.* 2006) gave placebo lozenges or *Streptococcus salivarius* K12 lozenges after a chlorhexidine mouthwash for three days. One week following the treatment, 85% of the probiotic group had substantially reduced (below 100 ppb) counts of halitosis-causing bacteria, while only 30% of the placebo group reached these levels.

An earlier study (Burton *et al.* 2005) found that in 8 out of 13 cases, reductions reached from *Streptococcus salivarius* K12 lozenges remained for two weeks after treatment.

Dry mouth: Hyposalivation or xerostomia often occurs among adults. The most prevalent cause of dry mouth is an increase in populations of oral yeasts (Shinozaki *et al.* 2012). These include the prolific *Candida albicans*, which we all harbor to some degree.

As discussed earlier, Candida and other yeast species are controlled by probiotic bacteria throughout the body. They are allowed to overgrow these regions when probiotic populations are decimated by our various antimicrobial measures.

Healthy probiotic populations can thus help relieve dry mouth.

In a Finnish study, 276 elderly persons suffering from oral Candida infections were given 50 grams of a probiotic-rich cheese daily or a non-probiotic cheese daily. After 16 weeks, the probiotic group experienced a 75% reduction in Candida yeast colonies, and a 56% reduction in dry mouth symptoms.

Respiratory Infections

There is sufficient evidence that pathogenic bacteria such as *Staphylococcus aureus, Streptococcus pneumoniae* and *Heomonphilus influenzae* can infect the lungs. Little research seems to have been done to confirm whether or not the lungs also harbor probiotic bacteria, however. Research has documented that probiotic bacteria inhabit the nasal cavity, the mouth and the throat. Research has also confirmed that ingested probiotics, probiotic lozenges and probiotic sprays can reduce lung infection incidence. Probiotics dwelling in the lungs or pleural cavity does not seem so radical: Certainly not as radical as the evidence showing intestinal probiotics can somehow inhibit bacteria in the upper respiratory tract.

Scientists from the Swiss National Accident Insurance Institute (Glück and Gebbers 2003) gave 209 human volunteers either a conventional yogurt or a combination of *Lactobacillus* GG (ATCC 53103), *Bifidobacterium* sp. B420, *Lactobacillus acidophilus* 145, and *Streptococcus thermophilus* every day for 3 weeks. Nasal microbial flora was measured at the beginning, at day 21 and at day 28 (a week after). Significant pathogenic bacteria were found in most of the volunteers' nasal cavities at the beginning of the study. The consumption of the probiotic-enhanced milk led to a 19% reduction of pathogenic bacteria in the nasal cavity. The researchers concluded that, *"The results indicate a linkage of the lymphoid tissue between the gut and the upper respiratory tract."*

Scientists from Barcelona (Cobo Sanz *et al.* 2006) gave 251 children aged 3 to 12 years milk either with or without *Lactobacillus casei* for 20 weeks. The probiotic group of children experienced significantly fewer respiratory tract infections, bronchitis and/or pneumonia (32% vs. 49%). The probiotic children also had a reduction in the duration of fatigue (3% vs. 13%). There was also a difference in the duration of sicknesses among the probiotic children compared to the placebo group.

French scientists (Forestier *et al.* 2008) assessed whether ventilator-associated pneumonia in intensive care units could be prevented or lessened by the use of probiotics. The 17-bed intensive care unit at the Clermont-Ferrand Teaching Hospital was used to test 208 patients with an intensive care unit stay of more than 48 hours. Patients were fed a placebo or *Lactobacillus rhamnosus* through a nasogastric feeding twice daily from their third day in the unit until discharge. Infective *Pseudomonas aeruginosa* cultures were measured at admission, once a week, and upon discharge. Bacteriological tests of the respiratory tract also were done to determine patient infections. The study results indicated that *P. aeruginosa* respiratory colonization and/or infection was significantly reduced among the probiotic group. Ventilator-associated pneumonia by *P. aeruginosa* in the probiotic group was reduced by more than 50% compared to the placebo group.

Researchers from the University of Arkansas' Medical School (Wheeler *et al.* 1997) studied 15 asthmatic adults in two 1-month crossover periods with placebo or yogurt containing *L. acidophilus*. The probiotic consumption increased immune system interferon gamma and decreased eosinophilia levels.

Greek scientists from the Faculty of Medicine of the University of Thessaloniki (Kotzampassi *et al.* 2006) gave a placebo or probiotic combination to 65 elderly critically ill, mechanically ventilated, multiple trauma patients for 15 days. The combination consisted of *Pediococcus pentosaceus* 5-33:3, *Leuconostoc mesenteroides* 32-77:1, *L. paracasei* subsp. *paracasei* 19; and *L. plantarum* 2,362; with inulin, oat bran, pectin and resistant starch as prebiotics. The probiotic patients had significantly lower levels of infection, sepsis and death than did the placebo group. Number of days in the ICU and number of days under ventilation were significantly reduced compared to the placebo group. The researchers concluded that: *"The administration of this synbiotic formula in critically ill, mechanically ventilated, multiple trauma patients seems to exert beneficial effects in respect to infection and sepsis rates and to improve the patient's response, thus reducing the duration of ventilatory support and intensive care treatment."*

Scientists from the University of Buenos Aires (Río *et al.* 2002) studied the incidence and severity of respiratory tract infections by giving 58 normal or undernourished children from 6 to 24 months old either a placebo or a combination of live *Lactobacillus acidophilus* and *Lactobacillus casei* probiotics. Their respiratory episodes were classified as pneumonia, bronchitis, recurrent obstructive bronchitis or upper respiratory tract infection. Total episodes in the probiotic group were 34; and 69 episodes occurred among the placebo group. The probiotic combination significantly suppressed pneumonia and bronchitis in both the normal and undernourished probiotic groups.

Rebuilding the Immune System

For some of us in the modern industrialized world, we have overloaded and burdened our immune systems to the point where we are suffering from constant inflammation, recurrent infection, allergies or autoimmunity. Probiotics have been shown to significantly reduce the incidence of these ailments. Probiotics are nature's smart army corps of engineers. Research has shown that they will help rebuild cellular functions and immune cell function, and help stimulate better immune system responses.

Furthermore, some of the research has confirmed that somehow, probiotics are able to stimulate the effects of vaccines. How are they able to do that? Remember that probiotics are living organisms that inhibit pathogens entering the body. As they do this, they can assist the immune system by stimulating specific immune responses. This means that probiotics retain a memory of pathogens, much as memory T-cells and B-cells do.

In the case of a vaccine, the vaccine is a small quantity of the pathogen itself, which stimulates the immune system to develop strategies to attack and rid the body of that pathogen should it invade the body later. Because probiotics help identify and stimulate immune responses, researchers have found that vaccination is often more productive when it is done concurrent to probiotic supplementation.

In a German study (de Vrese *et al.* 2005), 64 volunteers took either probiotics (*Lactobacillus rhamnosus* GG or *Lactobacillus acidophilus* CRL431) or placebo for five weeks. During the second week of treatment, the volunteers were given oral vaccinations against poliovirus 1, 2 and 4. As reported in other research, polio vaccination—even as documented by Dr. Salk—has caused on occasion the contraction of polio. Poliovirus factors—evident from poliovirus neutralizing antibody titers—increased significantly with probiotic treatment in this study. Increased vaccination response with probiotics ranged from two- to four-times higher. Furthermore, serum levels of *poliovirus-specific* IgA and IgG antibodies were significantly increased in the probiotic group. The researchers concluded that, *"Probiotics induce an immunologic response that may provide enhanced systemic protection of cells from virus infections by increasing production of virus neutralizing antibodies."*

Researchers from France's Université de Picardie (Mullié *et al.* 2004) gave 30 infants aged zero to four months poliovirus vaccinations along with a formula with *B. longum* and *B. infantis* or a placebo. In the probiotic group, antipoliovirus IgA responses significantly increased among the probiotic group versus the placebo group that received the vaccinations without probiotics. Antibody titers correlated with bifidobacteria levels, especially with *B. longum/B. infantis* and *B. breve* supplementation doses. The researchers were puzzled by the mechanism, adding, *"Whether this effect on the immune system is achieved through the bifidogenic effect of the formula (mainly through B. longum/B. infantis and B. breve stimulation) or directly linked to compounds (i.e. peptides) produced by milk fermentation remains to be investigated."*

Scientists from Finland's University of Turku (Fang *et al.* 2000) gave *Lactobacillus* GG, *Lactococcus lactis* or placebo to 30 healthy volunteers for 7 days. On the first, third and fifth days, a *Salmonella typhi* Ty21 oral vaccine was given to each volunteer to mimic enteropathogenic infection. A greater increase in specific IgA was observed among the *Lactobacillus* GG group. Among the *L. lactis* group, significantly higher CR3 receptor expression on neutrophils was observed compared to the placebo or *Lactobacillus* GG groups. The researchers concluded that, *"the immunomodulatory effect of probiotics is strain-dependent."*

Scientists from Finland's University of Tampere (Isolauri *et al.* 1995) studied the administration of *Lactobacillus* GG with oral rotavirus vaccines given to 2-5-month-old infants. Infants receiving the probiotic displayed an increased level of rotavirus-specific IgM secreting cells. The researchers concluded that, *"these findings suggest that LGG has an immunostimulating effect on oral rotavirus vaccination."*

Rebuilding the immune system with probiotics will return to the system the most vital part of preventing opportunistic infections: acquired immunity.

Illustrating this, Japanese scientists (Hirose *et al.* 2006) gave *Lactobacillus plantarum* strain L-137 or placebo to 60 healthy men and women, average age 56, for twelve weeks. Increased Con A-induced proliferation (acquired immunity), increases in IL-4 production by CD4+ T-cells, and a more balanced Th1:Th2 ratio was seen in the probiotic group. Quality of life criteria were also higher among the probiotic group.

Researchers from Britain's Scarborough Hospital (McNaught *et al.* 2005) gave a placebo or *Lactobacillus plantarum* 299v to 103 critically ill patients along with conventional therapy. On day 15, the probiotic group had significantly lower serum IL-6 levels compared to the control group.

Researchers from the Department of Immunology at Japan's Juntendo University School of Medicine (Takeda *et al.* 2006) gave a placebo or *Lactobacillus casei* Shirota to 9 healthy middle-aged adults and 10 elderly adults daily for three weeks. After three weeks of supplementation, *L. casei* significantly increased natural killer cell activity among the volunteers, especially among those who had low NK-cell activity before probiotic supplementation.

Researchers from the University of Vienna (Meyer *et al.* 2007) gave healthy women yogurt with starters *Lactobacillus bulgaricus* and *Streptococcus thermophilus*, with or without *Lactobacillus casei*. After two weeks, both yogurt groups had significantly increased blood levels of tumor necrosis factor-alpha (TNF-a): by 24% with the regular yogurt and by 63% with the *L. casei* yogurt. They also observed significantly higher levels of cytokines interleukin (IL)-1beta (by 40%) and interferon gamma (by 108%). In addition, IL-10 decreased during *L. casei*-enhanced yogurt treatment, but then significantly increased after the yogurt treatment was stopped (by 129%).

French scientists (Paineau *et al.* 2008) gave 83 healthy volunteers a placebo or seven probiotic strains, and tested their resulting antibody levels and immune response rates. IgG levels increased in the *Bifidobacterium lactis* Bl-04 and *Lactobacillus acidophilus* La-14 groups; and serum immunoglobulin levels increased significantly from six of the seven probiotic strains tested.

The bottom line is that probiotics stimulate and activate the immune system in numerous ways. They are in fact one of the most productive and important aspects of our immune system. They directly counteract invading microorganisms while stimulating the activities of immunoglobulins, T-cells and B-cells. Without sufficient probiotic colonies, our body's immune system is left severely handicapped.

Meet Your Oral Bacteria

More than 700 different species inhabit the mouth, nasal cavity, throat and lungs. Of these only 30-70 will dominate. Others will commingle in cooperative roles, managed by the more dominant species. These kinds of numbers might seem intimidating, but territorial domination keeps the various colonies well heeled.

Species and Strains

The two most important genera of oral probiotics are *Lactobacillus* and *Streptococcus.* Others include *Eubacterium, Fusobacterium, Peptococcaceae* and *Rheumanococcus.* Of these and others, our bodies each house a unique collection of species and strains.

These names may seem odd, but the nomenclature of genera, species and strains provides a common system for identification among scientists of different languages and parts of the world. This Latin-based naming system allows us to group species and strains, yet easily discern subtle differences between them. Species names often reflect a microorganism's respective activities, effects, cell appearance and other characteristics. Sometimes a name will reflect a disease or the environment from which it was discovered.

The strain name will further distinguish one organism from another. A strain name may describe the culture medium, the laboratory, and even the researchers who isolated the strain.

Large genetic differences can exist between different strains of the same probiotic bacteria species. Various *L. acidophilus* strains can differ up to 20% genetically, for example. Hundreds of strains have been found for some species. Over two decades ago, more than 200 strains of *L. acidophilus* had been isolated. Today this number has undoubtedly grown. The bottom line is that strains are often unique to each of us. A particular strain may colonize profusely in one person, and not in another.

Note that there are numerous probiotic subspecies strains that have been either isolated from different substrates or otherwise modified by scientists and commercial entities. There is evidence that some of these strains may be more vigorous than other strains of that species. However, conclusive evidence that these strains are necessarily more effective than *every* other strain of the same species has not been accomplished. Rigorous controlled, randomized and extensive studies would be required to confirm this possibility. It may well be that what might make one strain stronger than another is not necessarily the strain, but the special fermentation medium in which the strain was cultured. A unique culture is likely to produce unique characteristics among any strain of the same species simply because those organisms thriving in that culture become distinctive.

We might compare this to the differences between societies of people. A culture that thrived in the desert will have different strengths and weaknesses from one that thrived in the arctic. If we were stranded in the desert, we would likely want to have an Southwestern Indian as a companion rather than an Alaskan, for example.

Research focusing on particular patented strains is not such a bad thing, however. It has enabled commercial interests to fund research on probiotics—which has promoted the science of probiotics in numerous ways. We should be appreciative for the research, and have no issue buying their products with these possibly stronger strains. They also do not offer any significant restrictions to others who want to utilize the basic species or subspecies strains, either. Everyone is a winner in this sort of research.

At the same time, we should not dismiss strains that are not patented. A number of experts feel that non-patented strains of the same species can be just as potent as the patented strains.

Let's review the effects and characteristics of probiotics that have beneficial effects upon the oral, pharyngeal or nasal cavities, or the upper respiratory system in general.

The Bad and Not So Bad Guys

Here is a survey of some of the bacteria that have been shown to colonize within the mouth, upper respiratory tract and other regions. While some of these may be considered pathogenic in larger colonies, they may also be part of the biotic balance that exists within the body, and are therefore necessary to maintain health.

Actinobacillus actinomycetemcomitans

These bacteria infect gum pockets, and found in aggressive periodontitis. They are gram-negative, and produce endotoxins called leukotoxins, which damage blood cells and arteries.

Actinomyces sp.

These bacteria will live within the mouth and the pharynx. They are tiny bacteria, and are prevalent in soils, plants, and animals. They are known to be cooperative with various other bacteria, both probiotic and pathogenic. Working in combination with *Streptomyces*, for example, *Actinomyces* sp. can produce antibiotics such as actinomycin.

Clostridium sp.

These bacteria will typically inhabit the lower intestines and colon, although they may also inhabit the mouth and pharynx. Some of the more common species include *Clostridium difficile, Clostridium tetani,* and *Clostridium perfringens.* They are often implicated in various intestinal disorders.

Corynebacterium sp.

These bacteria are hardy and will inhabit the skin surfaces, the mouth, the nasal cavity, the pharynx, the conjunctiva of the eyes, the lower intestines and the vagina. Some species have been implicated in acne. *Corynebacterium diphtheriae* is quite common in the intestines, even to the point of being considered part of our healthy flora. When their populations become too large, however, they can cause a number of disease conditions, including diphtheria.

Entamoeba gingivalis

This protozoan is found in practically every case of periodontitis. They will inhabit the gum pockets. As their colonies grow, they can translocate to the throat and airways. They will readily destroy blood cells. Their endotoxins damage arteries, bones and other tissues.

Enterococcus faecalis (formerly *Streptococcus faecalis*)

These mostly pathogenic bacteria are normal residents of even healthy intestines. They can also dwell within the mouth, pharynx, urethra and vagina. They balance and strengthen our probiotics when in reasonable numbers. In larger numbers, however, they can be the cause for a number of diseases. Like other bacteria, several strains of *Enterococcus faecalis* have become antibiotic-resistant in recent years.

Escherichia coli and other *Enterobacteriaceae*

Enterobacteriaceae such as *E. coli* and *Proteus* sp. may dwell and thrive in the mouth, the nasal cavity, the pharynx, the eye conjunctiva, skin surfaces, the intestinal tract, the vagina and the urethra. *E. coli* are normal residents of most humans, but are still the source of disease when their populations grow. They have been known to be lethal in large populations. This illustrates the important role probiotics play in keeping populations of *E. coli* and other bacteria in control.

Haemophilus sp.

The *Haemophilus* genus contains several species that infect the mouth and airways. *H. influenzae* and is often the cause of a number of respiratory tract infections, especially among children. *H. aphrophilus* and *H. segnis* can infect the gums, producing periodontitis. They can also infect the eye conjunctiva and the colon and lower intestines. Many species are becoming resistant to antibiotics.

Helicobacter pylori

These bacteria are known to infect the stomach, causing ulcers, but they incubate in the mouth and expand in periodontitits. We discussed *H. pylori* in the last chapter, but what wasn't mentioned was that many *H. pylori* overgrowths come from oral infections.

Mycoplasmas

These microorganisms are known by their absence of a cell wall. They will commonly dwell in the lower intestines, the vagina, the mouth, the pharynx, and the urethra. One of the more pathogenic species is *Mycoplasma pneumoniae,* which are known to cause a disease referred to as walking pneumonia.

Neisseria meningitides

Neisseria meningitides bacteria inhabit primarily the pharynx, but will also live in the nasal cavity, the mouth and the vagina. These bacteria are the central cause for meningitis, which can be lethal. A combination of probiotics and an active immune system may readily control these bacteria, preventing serious infection while creating immunity to them.

Pseudomonas aeruginosa

These bacteria typically dwell on the skin, in the mouth, in the pharynx, in the walls of the urethra and within the colon. *P. aeruginosa* is hardy, and can live in oxygen and low-oxygen environments. *Pseudomonas aeruginosa* can infect wounds and enter through skin openings. They can cause lung infections, urinary tract infections and kidney infections. *Pseudomonas* has also been known to cause joint infections in a condition called septic arthritis.

Staphylococcus aureus

Most of us house these bacteria as normal residents. When controlled, they present little or no danger. They can live on skin surfaces, in the nose, mouth, vagina, ipharynx and intestines. They are not probiotic. However, as they compete with probiotics for territory, they strengthen the body's probiotics. Many strains of *Staphylococcus aureus* are extremely pathogenic, however, especially antibiotic-resistant strains such as MRSA. Aggressive *S. aureus* can become flesh eating should it be allowed to grow out of control on tissue surfaces. *S. aureus* can be one of the most aggressive and dangerous bacteria within an immunosuppressed body with depleted probiotic colonies. Other bacteria will co-habit tissues alongside staph, making staph infections even tougher to treat.

Staphylococcus epidermidis

These hardy probiotic or eubiotic organisms live on most of the body's epithelial surfaces. They thrive in the nasal cavity, in the pharynx, on the skin, in the conjunctiva of the eyes, in the lower urethra, in the vagina and in the colon and lower intestines. In the right colony numbers, *Staphylococcus epidermidis* can aggressively protect our skin and other membranes. *Staphylococcus epidermidis* will also adapt to varying temperatures and moisture content. They will also produce unique territorial acids that provide a protective layer for our skin and membrane surfaces. This protective acidic layer repels toxins, other bacteria, fungi and viruses.

Streptococcus mitis

These bacteria live primarily within the oral cavity and the pharynx. *Streptococcus mitis* are fairly normal residents of a healthy human body and help balance probiotic colonies. However, they can become pathogenic should they be allowed to outgrow our probiotic populations.

Streptococcus oralis

S. oralis are relatives of S. mitis, and are typical oral cavity inhabitants, and they are highly competitive. However, in sufficient numbers they can have a positive effect upon the airways, as they produce neuraminidase—which controls the spread of influenza. Some commercial research evidence has shown that S. oralis may also provide some teeth whitening as well.

Streptococcus pyrogenes

These bacteria dwell primarily within the oral cavity, the pharynx, the vagina, the conjunctiva of the eyes, and on the surface of the skin. They may also inhabit the intestines, but to a lesser degree. These bacteria are the central cause for strep throat and tonsillitis. Streptococcus pyrogenes can also cause pneumonia, rheumatic diseases, nephritis, and heart disease. They also stimulate inflammation, causing the swelling of tissues.

Streptococcus pneumoniae

These are fairly normal inhabitants of the respiratory tract. They also can live within the mouth, the vagina, the pharynx, and the nasal cavity. Streptococcus pneumoniae are the central cause for most cases of pneumonia. About 50% of the human population is thought to have S. pneumoniae inhabitants within the upper respiratory tract. This means that for those who have not contracted pneumonia, these populations are likely under control. This is the case for numerous organisms. While we have been taught to avoid them at all costs, in reality many of us host all or many of them. In a healthy body, colonies of territorial probiotics, with the help of the immune system, keep them managed.

Streptococcus mutans

S. mutans thrive primarily in the oral cavity and pharynx. These bacteria are the central cause for plaque formation around the teeth, and the main cause for dental caries and periodontal disease. S. mutans secrete acids that break down the enamel of our teeth, which causes cavities. They also thrive off simple starches and sugars. This is the reason that refined sugars and simple carbohydrates are known to cause cavities.

A relative of *S. mutans, Streptococcus rattus* (JH145) has been recently discovered by Dr. Jeffrey Hillman. This bacteria comingles and competes with *S. mutans,* yet produces no lactic acid—the cause for dental caries as we've discussed (Hillman *et al.* 2009). This new bacteria is now available in supplement form.

Treponema Denticola

These corkscrew-shaped bacteria (also called spirochetes) will inhabit available root canals and gum pockets. They are often found in gingivitis and periodontal disease. They produce endotoxins that can damage arteries and other tissues.

The Good Guys

Probiotic Streptococci

Bacteria from the genus Streptococcus play an important role in both disease and disease prevention. This is because when some species of *Streptococcus* become dominant, they will cause disease. In this scenario, some species of streptococci are quite aggressive and can cause lethal infections. A number of strains have also become antibiotic-resistant. Streptococci of different species and strains will inhabit the oral, nasal and pharyngeal cavities, as well as the intestines and other regions. They also produce a variety of bacteriocins that act as antibiotics to repel and kill other microorganisms. Here we will focus primarily upon the two dominant and related species, *Streptococcus salivarius* and *Streptococcus thermophilus.*

Streptococcus salivarius

Streptococcus salivarius are vigorous probiotic bacteria that station themselves throughout the upper respiratory tract, but primarily inhabit the oral cavity and pharynx. *S. salivarius* are the primary and most aggressive of our oral cavity probiotic bacteria. They are extremely territorial, and produce a number of antibiotics, including salivaricin A and salivaricin B, along with a host of other antibiotic substances.

They are also permanent residents in the human body. Our resident strains are inherited from mom. Mama transfers her resident strains through a combination of birthing, breast milk and kissing; although kissing and breast milk are likely the primary means. *Streptococcus salivarius* are extremely aggressive and will be the dominant species in a healthy mouth. This means that *Streptococcus salivarius* are organizers. To do this, they produce a number of enzymes and acids that manage the growth of other bacteria. One might conclude that *Streptococcus salivarius* are one of the most important bacteria to maintaining the health of the body, because they are the principal gatekeepers when it comes to preventing the entry and survival of infective microorganisms. As mentioned above, one of the mechanisms *S. Salivarius* utilize is the production of salivaricin. Salivaricin is recognized as one of the most potent group of antibiotics. While salivaricin A and salivaricin B have been isolated, it is certain that *S. salivarius* are constantly adjusting their antibiotic biochemistry to match new infective agents and their respective weaknesses.

Human clinical research has shown that *S. salivarius* can:
- ❖ Reduce dental plaque
- ❖ Reduce dental caries
- ❖ Inhibit gingivitis
- ❖ Inhibit *Streptococcus pyrogenes* (and strep throat)
- ❖ Prevent mastitis among breast-feeding mothers
- ❖ Reduce ulcerative colitis

Streptococcus thermophilus

Streptococcus thermophilus are considered subspecies of *S. salivarius*. Not surprisingly, *Streptococcus thermophilus* have been known to benefit the immune system in a number of ways. *Streptococcus thermophilus* are also commonly used in yogurt making. They are also used in cheese making, and are even sometimes found in pasteurized milk. They will colonize at higher temperatures, from 104-113 degrees F. This is significant because this bacterium readily produces lactase, which breaks down lactose. These are the only known streptococci that do this. Like other supplemented probiotics, *S. thermophilus* are temporary microorganisms in the human body. Their colonies will typically inhabit the system for a week or two before exiting. During that time, however, they will help set up a healthy environment to support resident colony growth. Like other probiotics, *S. thermophilus* also produce a number of different antibiotic substances and acids that deter the growth of pathogenic microorganisms.

Human clinical research has shown that *S. thermophilus* can:

- ❖ Reduce acute diarrhea (rotavirus and non-rotavirus)
- ❖ Reduce intestinal permeability
- ❖ Inhibit *H. pylori*
- ❖ Help manage AIDS symptoms
- ❖ Increase lymphocytes among low-WBC patients
- ❖ Increase IL-1beta
- ❖ Decrease IL-10
- ❖ Increase tumor necrosis factor-alpha (TNF-a)
- ❖ Increase absorption of dairy
- ❖ Decrease symptoms of IBS
- ❖ Inhibit *Clostridium difficile*
- ❖ Increase immune function among the elderly
- ❖ Restore infant microflora similar to breast-fed infants
- ❖ Increase CD8+
- ❖ Increase IFN-gamma
- ❖ Reduce acute gastroenteritis (diarrhea)
- ❖ Reduce baby colic
- ❖ Reduce symptoms of atopic dermatitis
- ❖ Reduce nasal cavity infections
- ❖ Increase HDL-cholesterol
- ❖ Increase growth in preterm infants
- ❖ Reduce intestinal bacteria
- ❖ Reduce upper respiratory tract infections from *Staphylococcus aureus*, *Streptococcus pneumoniae*, beta-hemolytic streptococci, and *Haemophilus influenzae*
- ❖ Increase HDL cholesterol
- ❖ Reduce urine oxalates (kidney stones)
- ❖ Reduce *S. mutans* in the mouth
- ❖ Reduce flare-ups of chronic pouchitis
- ❖ Reduce LDL-cholesterol in overweight subjects
- ❖ Reduce ulcerative colitis

The Lactobacilli

Lactis means "milk" in Latin. Lactobacilli are primarily found in the small intestines, although they will also inhabit the oral cavity, the nasal cavity, and the pharynx. Lactobacilli lower the pH of their environment by converting long-chain saccharides (complex sugars) such as lactose to lactic acid. This conversion process effectively inhibits pathogen growth and creates the appropriate acidic environment for other probiotics to colonize.

Lactobacillus salivarius

Lactobacillus salivarius are typical residents of most humans— although supplemented versions will still be transients. They are also found in the intestines of other animals. L. salivarius will dwell in the mouth, the nasal cavity, the pharynx, the small intestines, the colon, and the vagina. They are hardy bacteria that can live in both oxygen and oxygen-free environments. L. salivarius is one of the few bacteria species that can also thrive in salty environments. They can also survive many medications.

L. salivarius produce prolific amounts of lactic acid, which makes them hardy defenders of the teeth and gums. They also produce a number of antibiotics, and are speedy colonizers. Upon ingestion, they quickly combat pathogenic bacteria and defend their territory. Because of their hardiness, they will readily take out massive numbers of pathogens immediately. L. salivarius are also known to be able to break apart complex proteins.

Human clinical research has shown that Lactobacillus salivarius can:
- ❖ Inhibit S. mutans in the mouth
- ❖ Reduce dental carries
- ❖ Reduce gingivitis and periodontal disease
- ❖ Reduce mastitis
- ❖ Reduce risk of strep throat caused by S. pyogenes
- ❖ Reduce ulcerative colitis and IBS
- ❖ Inhibit E. coli
- ❖ Inhibit Salmonella spp.
- ❖ Inhibit Candida albicans

Lactobacillus reuteri

L. reuteri is a species found residing permanently in humans. As a result, most supplemented strains attach to mucosal membranes, though temporarily, and stimulate the colony growth of resident L. reuteri strains. L. reuteri will colonize in the oral cavity, the nasal cavity, and the pharynx, stomach, duodenum and ileum regions. L. reuteri will also significantly modulate the immune response of the gastrointestinal mucosal membranes. This means that L. reuteri are effective for many of the same digestive ailments that L. acidophilus are used for. L. reuteri also have several other effects, including the restoration of our oral cavity bacteria. They also produce a significant amount of antibiotic biochemicals.

Human clinical research has shown that *L. reuteri* can:
- ❖ Inhibit gingivitis
- ❖ Reduce pro-inflammatory cytokines
- ❖ Help re-establish the pH of the vagina
- ❖ Stimulate growth and feeding among preterm infants
- ❖ Inhibit and suppress *H. pylori*
- ❖ Decrease dyspepsia
- ❖ Increase CD3+ in HIV patients
- ❖ Reduce nausea
- ❖ Reduce flatulence
- ❖ Reduce diarrhea (rotavirus and non-rotavirus)
- ❖ Reduce TGF-beta2 in breast-feeding mothers (reduced risk of eczema)
- ❖ Reduce *Streptococcus mutans*
- ❖ Stimulate the immune system
- ❖ Reduce plaque on teeth
- ❖ Inhibit vaginal candidiasis
- ❖ Decrease symptoms of IBS
- ❖ Increase CD4+ and CD25 T-cells in IBS
- ❖ Decrease TNF-alpha in IBS patients
- ❖ Decrease IL-12 in IBS
- ❖ Reduce IgE eczema in infancy
- ❖ Reduce infant colic
- ❖ Restore vagina pH
- ❖ Reduce colds and influenza
- ❖ Stabilize intestinal barrier function (reducing intestinal permeability)
- ❖ Decrease atopic dermatitis

Lactobacillus acidophilus

Lactobacillus acidophilus are by far the most familiar probiotic bacteria to most of us, and are also by far the most-studied to date. They are one of the main residents of the human gut, although supplemented strains will still be transient. They are also found in the mouth and vagina. *L. acidophilus* grow best in warm (85-100 degrees F) and moist environments. Many are facultative anaerobic, meaning they can grow in oxygen-rich or oxygen-poor environments. *L. acidophilus* bacteria were first discovered by Ilya Metchnikoff in the first decade of the twentieth century. Within a few years, *L. acidophilus* remedies were found in many venues, but they were poorly handled because many did not understand how easily probiotics would die outside of the intestines. Then in the late 1940s, scientists from the University of Nebraska began focused studies on *Lactobacillus acidophilus* to determine how to produce them, maintain them, and supply them as medicines.

Probably the most important benefit of *L. acidophilus* is their ability to inhibit the growth of pathogenic microorganisms, not only in the gut, but also throughout the body. *L. acidophilus* significantly control and rid the body of *Candida albicans* overgrowth, which can invade various tissues of the body if unchecked. They also inhibit *Escherichia coli*, which can be fatal in large enough populations. They can also inhibit the growth of *Helicobacter pylori*—implicated in ulcers; *Salmonella*—a genus of deadly infectious bacteria; and *Shigella* and *Staphylococcus*—both potentially lethal infectious bacteria. It should be noted that *L. acidophilus'* ability to block these infectious agents will depend upon the size of the pathobiotic colonization and the size of the *L. acidophilus* colonies. *L. acidophilus* produces a variety of antibiotic substances, including acidolin, acidophillin, lactobacillin, lactocidin and others.

L. acidophilus lessen pharmaceutical antibiotic side effects; aid lactose absorption; help the absorption of various nutrients; help maintain the mucosa; help balance the pH of the upper intestinal tract; create a hostile environment for invading yeasts; and inhibit urinary tract and vaginal infections.

L. acidophilus also produce several digestive enzymes, including lactase, lipase and protease. Lactase is an enzyme that breaks down lactose. Several studies have shown that milk- or lactose-intolerant people are able to handle milk once they have established colonies of *L. acidophilus*. Lypase helps break down fatty foods, and protease helps break down protein foods.

Human clinical research indicates that *L. acidophilus* can:
- ❖ Lower LDL and total cholesterol
- ❖ Help digest milk
- ❖ Increase growth rates
- ❖ Reduce stress-induced GI problems
- ❖ Inhibit *E. coli*
- ❖ Reduce infection from rotavirus
- ❖ Reduce necrotizing enterocolitis
- ❖ Reduce intestinal permeability
- ❖ Control *H. pylori*
- ❖ Modulate PGE2 and IgA
- ❖ Reduce dyspepsia
- ❖ Modulate IgG
- ❖ Relieve and inhibit IBS and colitis
- ❖ Inhibit keratoconjunctivitis (in eye drops)

- ❖ Inhibit and control *Clostridium* spp.
- ❖ Inhibit *Bacteroides* spp.
- ❖ Inhibit and resolve acute diarrhea
- ❖ Reduce vaginosis and vaginitis
- ❖ Decrease triglycerides
- ❖ Increase appetite
- ❖ Increase growth in preterm infants
- ❖ Inhibit *Candida* spp. overgrowths
- ❖ Produce B vitamins and other nutrients
- ❖ Reduce anemia
- ❖ Increase vaccine efficiency
- ❖ Produce virus-specific antibodies
- ❖ Reduce allergic response
- ❖ Reduce urinary oxalate levels
- ❖ Inhibit antibiotic-related diarrhea
- ❖ Decrease allergic symptoms
- ❖ Inhibit upper respiratory infections
- ❖ Increase (good) HDL-cholesterol
- ❖ Inhibit tonsillitis
- ❖ Reduce blood pressure
- ❖ Inhibit viruses
- ❖ Increase leukocytes
- ❖ Increase calcium absorption

Lactobacillus helveticus

L. helveticus is a probiotic species made popular in Switzerland. Latin *Helvetia* refers to the country of Switzerland. *L. helveticus* is used in cheese making. *L. helveticus* is used as starter bacteria for Swiss cheese and several other cheeses. *L. helveticus* will also inhabit the oral cavity temporarily as these cheeses are eaten. *L. helveticus* grow optimally between 102 and 122 degrees F. One of the reasons *L. helveticus* are favored cheese starters is because they produce primarily lactic acid and fewer metabolites, which can make the cheese taste bitter or sour.

Human clinical research has shown that *L. helveticus* can:
- ❖ Reduce blood pressure among hypertensive patients
- ❖ Produce ACE-inhibitor molecules
- ❖ Increase sleep quality and duration
- ❖ Increase general health perception
- ❖ Increase serum levels of calcium
- ❖ Decrease PTH (parathyroid hormone—marker for bone loss)
- ❖ Normalize gut colonization similar to breast-fed infants among formula-fed infants

Lactobacillus casei

L. casei are typically transient bacteria that will inhabit the mouth, pharynx, nasal cavity and intestines. They are commonly used in a number of food applications and industrial applications. These include culturing cheese and other milk products, and fermenting green olives. *L. casei* is found naturally in raw milk and in colostrum—meaning they are typical residents of cows. *L. casei* have been reported to reduce allergy symptoms and increase immune response. This seems to be accomplished by regulating the immune system's CHS, CD8 and T-cell responsiveness. However, this immune stimulation seems to be evident primarily among immunosuppressed patients (Guerin-Danan *et al.* 1998). This of course is an indication that probiotics can somehow uniquely respond to the host's particular condition. Some strains of *L. casei* are also very aggressive, and within a mixed probiotic supplement or food, they can dominate and even remove other bacteria.

Human clinical research has shown that *L. casei* can:
- ❖ Inhibit pathogenic bacterial infections
- ❖ Reduce occurrence, risk and symptoms of IBS
- ❖ Inhibit severe systemic inflammatory response syndrome
- ❖ Decrease C-reactive protein (CRP)
- ❖ Inhibit pneumonia
- ❖ Inhibit respiratory tract infections
- ❖ Inhibit bronchitis
- ❖ Maintain remission of diverticular disease
- ❖ Inhibit *H. pylori* (and ulcers)
- ❖ Reduce allergy symptoms
- ❖ Inhibit *Pseudomonas aeruginosa*
- ❖ Decrease milk intolerance
- ❖ Increase CD3+ and CD4+
- ❖ Increase phagocytic activity
- ❖ Support liver function
- ❖ Decrease risk of cirrhosis
- ❖ Decrease cytokine TNF-alpha
- ❖ Stimulate the immune system
- ❖ Inhibit and reduce diarrhea episodes
- ❖ Produce vitamins B1 and B2
- ❖ Prevent recurrence of bladder cancer
- ❖ Stimulate cytokine interleukin-1beta (IL-1b)
- ❖ Stimulate interferon-gamma
- ❖ Inhibit *Clostridium difficile*
- ❖ Reduce asthma symptoms
- ❖ Reduce constipation

- ❖ Decrease beta-glucuronidase (associated with colon cancer)
- ❖ Stimulate natural killer cell activity (NK-cells)
- ❖ Increase IgA levels
- ❖ Increase lymphocytes
- ❖ Decrease IL-6 (pro-inflammatory)
- ❖ Increase IL-12 (stimulates NK-cells)
- ❖ Reduce lower respiratory infections
- ❖ Inhibit *Candida* overgrowth
- ❖ Inhibit vaginosis
- ❖ Prevent colorectal tumor growth
- ❖ Restore NK-cell activity in smokers
- ❖ Stimulate the immune system among the elderly
- ❖ Increase oxygen burst activity of monocytes
- ❖ Increase CD56 lymphocytes
- ❖ Decrease rotavirus infections
- ❖ Decrease colds and influenza
- ❖ Reduce risk of bladder cancer
- ❖ Increase (good) HDL-cholesterol
- ❖ Decrease triglycerides
- ❖ Decrease blood pressure
- ❖ Inhibit viral infections
- ❖ Inhibit malignant pleural effusions secondary to lung cancer
- ❖ Reduce cervix tumors when used in combination radiation therapy
- ❖ Inhibit tumor growth of carcinomatous peritonitis/stomach cancer
- ❖ Break down nutrients for bioavailability

Lactobacillus rhamnosus

This species was previously thought to be a subspecies of *L. casei*. *L. rhamnosus* is a common ingredient in many yogurts and other commercial probiotic foods. *L. rhamnosus* have also been extensively studied over the years. Much of this research has focused upon a particular strain, *L. rhamnosus* GG. *L. rhamnosus* GG have been shown in numerous studies to significantly stimulate the immune system and inhibit a variety of infections. *L. rhamnosus* will also dwell in the mouth, pharynx and nasal cavity on a transient basis, but not for very long. This strain also has shown to have good intestinal wall adhesion properties. This is not to say, however, that non-GG strains will not perform similarly. In fact, studies with *L. rhamnosus* GR-1, *L. rhamnosus* 573/L, and *L. rhamnosus* LC705 strains have also showed positive results. The GG strain (LGG is trademarked by the Valio Ltd. Company in Finland) was patented in 1985 by two scientists, Dr. Sherwood Gorbach and Dr. Barry Goldin (hence the Gs). This patent and trademark, of course, gives these companies the incentive to fund expensive research to show the properties of this strain. Thanks to them, we have found that *Lactobacillus rhamnosus* (or the GG strain specifically) has a number of the health-promoting properties.

Human clinical research has shown that *L. rhamnosus* can:

- ❖ Inhibit a number of pathogenic bacterial infections
- ❖ Improve glucose control
- ❖ Reduce risk of ear infections
- ❖ Reduce risk of respiratory infections
- ❖ Decrease beta-glucosidase
- ❖ Inhibit vaginosis
- ❖ Reduce eczema
- ❖ Reduce colds and influenza
- ❖ Stimulate the immune system
- ❖ Increase IgA levels in mouth mucosa
- ❖ Increase IgA levels in mothers breast milk
- ❖ Inhibit *Pseudomonas aeruginosa* infections in respiratory tract
- ❖ Inhibit *Clostridium difficile*
- ❖ Increase immune response in HIV/AIDS patients
- ❖ Inhibit rotavirus
- ❖ Inhibit enterobacteria
- ❖ Reduce IBS symptoms
- ❖ Decrease IL-12, IL-2+ and CD69+ T-cells in IBS
- ❖ Reduce constipation
- ❖ Inhibit vancomycin-resistant enterococci (antibiotic-resistant)
- ❖ Reduce the risk of colon cancer
- ❖ Modulate skin IgE sensitization
- ❖ Inhibit *H. pylori* (ulcer-causing)
- ❖ Reduce atopic dermatitis in children
- ❖ Increase Hib IgG levels in allergy-prone infants
- ❖ Reduce colic
- ❖ Stimulate infant growth
- ❖ Stimulate IgM, IgA and IgG levels
- ❖ Stabilize intestinal barrier function (decreased permeability)
- ❖ Increase INF-gamma
- ❖ Modulate IL-4
- ❖ Help prevent atopic eczema
- ❖ Reduce *Streptococcus mutans*
- ❖ Stimulate tumor killing activity among NK-cells
- ❖ Modulate IL-10 (anti-inflammatory)
- ❖ Reduce inflammation
- ❖ Reduce LDL-cholesterol levels

Lactobacillus plantarum

L. plantarum has been part of the human diet for thousands of years, and will live in the mouth and the pharynx transiently, and the intestines on a longer-term basis. They are active in cultures of sauerkraut, gherkin and olive brines. They are used to make sourdough bread, Nigerian ogi and fufu, kocha from Ethiopia, and sour mifen noodles from China, Korean kim chi and other traditional foods. *L. plantarum* are also found in dairy and cow dung, so it is a common resident of cow intestines, which is one reason why cow dung is considered in India as being antiseptic.

L. plantarum is a hardy strain. The bacteria have been shown to survive all the way through the intestinal tract and into the feces. Temperature for optimal growth is 86-95 degrees F. *L. plantarum* are not permanent residents, however. When supplemented, they vigorously attack pathogenic bacteria, and create an environment hospitable for incubated resident strains to expand. *L. plantarum* also produce lysine, and a number of antibiotics including lactolin.
Human clinical research has shown that *L. plantarum* can:
- ❖ Reduce burn infections (topical)
- ❖ Increase burn healing
- ❖ Strengthen the immune system
- ❖ Help restore healthy liver enzymes (alcohol-induced liver injury)
- ❖ Reduce frequency and severity of respiratory diseases during the cold and flu season
- ❖ Reduce intestinal permeability
- ❖ Inhibit various intestinal pathobiotics (such as *Clostridium difficile*)
- ❖ Reduce Th2 (inflammatory) levels and increase Th1/Th2 ratio
- ❖ Reduce inflammatory responses
- ❖ Reduce symptoms and aid healing of multiple traumas among injured patients
- ❖ Reduce fungal infections
- ❖ Reduce IBS symptoms
- ❖ Reduce pancreatic sepsis (infection)
- ❖ Reduce systolic blood pressure
- ❖ Reduce leptin levels (good for weight loss)
- ❖ Reduce interleukin-6 (IL-6) levels
- ❖ Reduce adhesion of vein endothelial cells by monocytes (risk of atherosclerosis)
- ❖ Reduce postoperative infection
- ❖ Reduce risk of pneumonia
- ❖ Reduce kidney oxalate levels
- ❖ Decrease flatulence

❖ Stimulate immunity in HIV children

Lactobacillus bulgaricus

We owe the *bulgaricus* name to Ilya Mechnikov, who named it after the Bulgarians—who used *L. bulgaricus* to make the fermented milks that appeared to be related to their extreme longevity. In the 1960s and 1970s, Russian researcher Dr. Ivan Bogdanov focused on the secretions of *L. bulgaricus* and later on fragmented cell walls of the bacteria. Early studies indicated antitumor effects. As the research progressed into clinical research and commercialization, it became obvious that *L. bulgaricus* cell fragments have a host of immune system stimulating benefits.

L. bulgaricus bacteria are transients that assist *bifidobacteria* colony growth. *L. bulgaricus* stimulate the immune system and have antitumor effects. They also produce antibiotic and antiviral substances such as bulgarican and others. *L. bulgaricus* bacteria have been reported to have anti-herpes effects as well. *L. bulgaricus* require more heat to colonize than many probiotics—at 104-109 degrees F.

Human clinical research has shown that *L. bulgaricus* can:
- ❖ Reduce intestinal permeability
- ❖ Decrease IBS symptoms
- ❖ Help manage HIV symptoms
- ❖ Stimulate TNF-alpha
- ❖ Stimulate IL-1beta
- ❖ Decrease diarrhea (rotavirus and non-rotavirus)
- ❖ Decrease nausea
- ❖ Increase phagocytic activity
- ❖ Increase leukocyte levels
- ❖ Increase immune response
- ❖ Increase CD8+ levels
- ❖ Lower CD4+/CD8+ ratio (lower CD4+—associated with inflammation)
- ❖ Increase IFN-gamma
- ❖ Lower total cholesterol
- ❖ Lower LDL levels
- ❖ Lower triglycerides
- ❖ Inhibit viruses
- ❖ Reduce *S. mutans* in the mouth
- ❖ Increase absorption of dairy (lactose)
- ❖ Increase white blood cell counts after chemotherapy

- ❖ Increase IgA specific to rotavirus (increased immunity against rotavirus)
- ❖ Reduce intestinal bacteria

Lactobacillus brevis

L. brevis are natural residents of cow intestines. They are therefore found in raw milk, colostrum, and cheese. For those who consume these frequently, *L. brevis* will temporarily inhabit the oral cavity and pharynx. They are transient in humans, but there is also the possibility that they can reside longer-term or permanently within the human intestines.

Human clinical research has shown that *L. brevis* can:
- ❖ Reduce periodontal disease
- ❖ Reduce PGE2 levels
- ❖ Reduce IFN-gamma levels
- ❖ Reduce mouth ulcers
- ❖ Reduce urinary oxalate levels (kidney stones)
- ❖ Decrease *H. pylori* colonization

Oral Probiotic Supplements

Supplementation with oral probiotics consists of consuming a probiotic species or combination that will begin colonizing within the oral cavity. This type of supplementation will typically spread to the nasal cavity, the pharynx, and even sometimes into the respiratory tract with some time. Our discussion here will focus upon those supplements that allow for oral cavity colonization.

The pertinent question about oral cavity probiotic supplementation is how long they will survive. To answer this question, a study was conducted at the Department of Microbiology and Immunology at the University of Otago in Dunedin, New Zealand (Burton *et al.* 2005) on 14 young men and women (average age 19). Saliva was collected and tested a day prior to supplementation. After teeth brushing and a chlorhexidine mouthwash, each was given a lozenge with *Streptococcus salivarius* K12 every two hours for a period of eight hours. This was repeated daily for two more days. Saliva samples were drawn after three days, five days, fourteen days, and 28 days—25 days after supplementation ceased. Before supplementation with K12, only two had *S. salivarius* organisms that displayed K-12-like antibiotic (bacteria-killing) activities. After taking the K12 lozenges for two days, 13 out of 14 subjects' oral cavities contained *S. salivarius* colonies with this antibiotic activity. This number reduced to only four of the subjects after the 28 days (25 days after supplementation ceased). However, this K12-like antibacterial activity persisted among the other subjects for more than one month after supplementation ceased. Interestingly, total counts of *Streptococcus salivarius* and other probiotic bacteria remained about the same throughout the study, while colonies of *S. mutans, Pseudomonas, Candida,* coliforms and *Staphylococcus aureus* were reduced. In other words, while there was not a significant net increase in *Streptococcus salivarius* colonies, there was an increase in the K12-like antibacterial activity of all *S. salivarius* colonies (residents and supplemented) during and after the *S. salivarius* K12 supplementation. Furthermore, the tests showed that levels of the K12 decreased over the period of supplementation, even as antibacterial activity increased.

What does all this tell us about oral cavity probiotic supplementation? First it tells us that supplementation with the oral probiotic strains will stimulate antibiotic activity among our resident oral probiotics. Remember the plasmids? This would be the likely mechanism. Hardy supplemented strains are simply passing their antibiotic knowledge on to our resident strains.

This study also confirms that supplemented strains are typically transients. This is consistent with studies on intestinal probiotic supplementation. Intestinal probiotic supplement strains typically will remain for about two weeks after supplementation is discontinued. This study tells us that supplemented oral probiotics may remain for about the same period two weeks to a month perhaps, but during that time, they will stimulate antibiotic activity among the resident strains. This stimulation will outlast the supplemental period because the resident strains have inherited the information. This enhanced potential should remain as long as those activated probiotic colonies are supported and nurtured.

We should note that the above study only utilized probiotic supplements for three days. A typical course would be for several months, providing a more pronounced immunostimulatory effect.

Remember that large genetic differences can exist between different strains of the same probiotic species. Some strains may not colonize well in some people, while colonizing prolifically in others. This can depend upon our existing probiotic colonies, dietary choices, stress levels and other environmental issues.

Most supplemental probiotic species and strains have undergone significant research and testing for safety before they are packaged and sold commercially as supplements. Human-friendly strains are standardized, identified and cataloged within the *American Type Culture Collection* (ATCC) in Manassas, Virginia; or the *Collection Nationale de Cultures de Microorganismes* at the Institut Pasteur in France. The majority of probiotic supplements sold in the U.S. are (or should be) listed in the ATCC.

It should also be clarified that commercial strains do not always mimic those results found from researched strains. Researchers often uniquely culture a particular strain for the research. The particular culture technique may not equate to those culturing techniques being used for a specific brand's commercial production. Other research has used commercial strains, but even then, their handling within the study may not equate to how the commercial strain is handled by the manufacturers, distributors, stores and consumers of those strains. This is not to say that a supplemental probiotic will necessarily have fewer effects than one involved in clinical study. It may be that the commercial version may be handled in a manner superior to the researched version, and/or within an environment more conducive for the effects of that strain.

Oral Probiotic Supplement Options

Lozenges: Lozenges release probiotic colony forming units as they are being sucked on. As a result, lozenges have been the subject of numerous studies showing probiotics' successful colonization into the oral cavity and upper respiratory tract. The benefit of lozenges is that they release the probiotics very slowly as they gain contact with the moisture and heat of the mouth. This allows the early colonies to begin to build their lactic acid environment for the colonies released thereafter. This 'bootstraping' process allows for a greater total colonization, compared to introducing the entire supplement contents into the environment at the same time.

Chewing Gum: Several new probiotic gums have been recently introduced to the market. These can also provide a slower release of probiotics, albeit likely not as slowly as lozenges might. Gums will release their 'payload' as we chew on them, and depending upon our chewing technique, they can insert colonies into our gum line. The benefits of these gums also depend upon their additional ingredients. A gum with simple sugar sweeteners will provide food and energy for competitive pathogenic species, so this is not suggested. Probiotic gums with xylitol have been shown to be superior. Even xylitol gum without probiotics has been shown to have positive effects upon the gums and plaque.

Chewable tablets: There are now a few chewable tablets or wafers also available to the market. These are distinguished from long-time brands that offered chewable tablets or wafers of *Lactobacillus acidophilus* intended for the digestive tract within a chewable form. This is not to say that these *L. acidophilus* chewable tablets do not offer some benefit to our oral probiotic colonies. *L. acidophilus* do colonize within the mouth, but *L. reuteri, L. salivarius, S. salivarius, S. uberis, S. oralis* and/or *S. rattus* will be more aggressive towards pathogenic oral bacteria and supportive of oral probiotic growth.

Capsules: Freeze-dried probiotics in capsules are designed to completely bypass the oral cavity. These probiotic formulations are typically intended for delivery to the intestinal tract. This doesn't mean that we cannot just empty the capsule contents into our mouths and swish it around the mouth with a little water or milk. Capsule formulations, however, are not intended to colonize the oral cavity. They may be helpful temporarily in combating an oral infection in a pinch, but they may also crowd out some of the mouth's resident probiotics. Better to choose *L. reuteri, L. salivarius, S. salivarius, S. uberis, S. oralis and/or S. rattus* strains.

Powders: Like capsule contents, powders of freeze-dried probiotics may also be swished around the mouth to provide some colonization in the oral and nasal cavities. Again, these may or may not be designed for oral cavity supplementation.

Caplets, Tablets, Shells or Beads: These probiotics supplement formats are formulated and designed for intestinal delivery. While they may deliver probiotic colonies to the intestines and benefit our oral probiotics indirectly, they will likely not work for oral cavity supplementation. This said, in some cases (depending upon the strains) there could be a benefit to occasionally dissolving in the mouth, as they could deplete pathogenic colonies within the mouth and throat.

Liquid Supplements: There are a few liquid probiotic supplements that work well for oral cavity supplementation. They are not necessarily designed as such, but just as probiotic foods can deliver probiotics into the oral cavity, these liquid supplements can deliver colonies into the oral cavity with a little swishing around the mouth. One particular well-known brand uses a hardy strain of *L. reuteri,* which has been shown to have good effects in the oral, pharyngeal and nasal cavities.

Probiotic Foods: As mentioned, probiotic foods such as yogurt, kefir, buttermilk, cheeses and others can provide oral supplementation to the degree they are slowly chewed or swished around the mouth a little. This may be limited by the species within the probiotic food, and the handling and production of the probiotic food prior to its delivery to the mouth. Nonetheless, the swishing around the mouth of our favorite probiotic foods would not be a bad idea. We'll discuss some of these more specifically later on.

Dosage Considerations

Most experts agree that a good maintenance dose for intestinal probiotics is ten to fifteen billion CFU ("colony forming units") per day for adults. Double or triple those dosage levels is suggested during an illness or therapeutic period. Much of the clinical research utilized dosages in this therapeutic range and even higher.

Children's dosages would depend upon age. Consulting with a health practitioner educated in probiotic supplementation is suggested before dosing children with probiotics.

Supplemental oral cavity probiotic dosages are far less than intestinal dosages, especially when the formula contains the hardy *Lactobacillus reuteri, Streptococcus salivarius, S. uberis, S. oralis and/or S. rattus*. In this case, a dose of 100 million to 1 billion per day should be adequate. One of the reasons why fewer CFUs are needed to colonize the oral cavity is because oral probiotics are immediately delivered into the mouth. They are not met with a challenging environment prior to reaching their destination, as intestinal probiotics face with the stomach. They also easily propagate in the presence of saliva.

The best times for taking oral probiotics are at bedtime after brushing the teeth, or during the day after a meal and after brushing. Many commercial toothpastes are designed to remove bacteria, so they can hamper oral probiotic colonies. It is thus a good idea to rinse the mouth thoroughly with water after brushing before consuming oral probiotics.

In addition, sugary foods will promote the growth of the pathogenic competitors to our probiotics. Therefore, it is not a good idea to eat sugary foods after or during oral probiotic ingestion. This will allow probiotic bacteria to colonize with less resistance.

Travelers are advised to take intestinal probiotics before, after and while traveling to avoid infection from strange microbes in foreign food and water. Traveling with oral probiotics can also lower the risk of infection from breathing in pathogenic microorganisms on crowded buses or airplanes.

Oral Flora Residents

Most of the focus of five decades of research on probiotics has been upon intestinal probiotics. As a result, oral probiotic research has not gained much attention among the health media. Furthermore, the number of species inhabiting the mouth has been assumed small. In a 2005 study from the University of Oslo, Norway and the Harvard School of Dental Medicine (Aas *et al.* 2005) determined through the examination of five human subjects that up to 700 species of bacteria live amongst the tongue, the hard and soft palates, the gingival plaque on tooth surfaces, the maxillary anterior vestibule, and the tonsils. This amazing number of species illustrates just how complex the environment within the mouth is.

Consequently, oral probiotics deserve more focus and research. In fact, there is a lot that we don't know about microorganisms in general.

Research has shown that intestinal probiotic strains obtained from mama through the birthing canal, through mother's milk, kissing or other contact with mama become permanent residents of the intestinal tract. As Dr. Jeremy Burton's research illustrated earlier, this is also likely true of oral probiotics. Supplemented strains may establish some new activity amongst themselves and the resident strains, but in the end, the resident strains should resume their dominance in a healthy mouth.

Assuming conservative antibiotic intake and a relatively healthy diet, we should have plenty of healthy resident oral cavity colonies. This would be evidenced by fewer seasonal illnesses when others around us are ill with colds or influenza. In the western world, the average modern adult will likely have lost or depleted their resident strains with repeated doses of antibiotics, pollution, preservatives and other chemicals that can damage these important colonies.

These toxins will weaken our resident populations, opening them up to being overrun by pathogenic microorganisms. As our probiotic strains become weakened by diet and toxicity, aggressive transients or pathogenic residents move in to take their places. This doesn't mean our resident probiotics become extinct, however. They may be present in smaller numbers, but controlled by the larger pathogenic populations.

The research has shown that supplemented versions of the more aggressive *L. reuteri, L. salivarius* and/or *S. salivarius* species can successfully decrease populations of pathogenic microorganisms. They can then help set up a suitable environment for our resident strains to re-emerge and regain control.

Where might they re-emerge from? Again they may well be present but in smaller colony counts within the oral cavity. If they are more thoroughly reduced by antibiotics, the Duke University study (Randal, *et al.* 2007) discussed earlier illustrated that the lymphatic system—more specifically the appendix—may incubate some remaining resident strains. We might compare this to a bomb shelter or a seed vault.

As we extend this finding to the observation that mother's breast milk contains up to 40% resident probiotics and immunoglobulins by volume and the mammary glands connect to the lymphatic system, it seems logical to conclude that other lymphatic nodes also incubate resident probiotic strains. The tonsils and lymph nodes that gather around the pharynx may incubate resident probiotic strains, for example.

After all, both the appendix and the tonsils swell in the face of infection. Both are part of the lymphatic system. Both are in regions that are central passageways for toxins and bacteria. It would only be logical if both also served the same purpose of incubating resident probiotic strains, as the appendix was found to do. Certainly, we have little alternative reason for the existence of the tonsils. It has appeared quite useless to medical researchers. Like the tonsils, the appendix has not been considered necessary. As a result, surgical removal of both is quite common.

Doctors may well be handicapping the future immunity of the patient by casually removing these important parts of the immune system. Studies have indeed confirmed a number of immunological changes occur within patients that have their tonsils removed. A Japanese study several decades ago (Yamauchi et al. 1981) confirmed that Hodgkin's disease risk was tripled following tonsillectomy. Other more recent studies indicate immediate changes in immune factors such as CD4+ and CD25+ (Kaygusuz et al. 2003). More studies are needed to confirm this, but it is logical to assume that probiotic incubation occurs within the tonsils.

As for intestinal probiotics, research has indicated that the probiotic colonies that propagate our digestive tracts and oral cavity in our first 6-18 months are the ones that stay with us throughout our lives. These will grow within our digestive tracts and become recognized by our immune systems. They will also harbor deep within the mucoid plaque along the walls of our digestive tract and congregate in our oral cavity, nasal cavity and pharynx. Should we knock out thriving colonies with antibiotics, chemicals or toxins, our resident strains may still be able to colonize and grow, assuming we re-establish the right environment for them.

This tells us that resident strains of probiotics are primarily those that have cultured within our families, and are a genetic match for our bodies. The probiotic strains that we receive from our mothers are likely the same strains that we will pass on to our children. Just as our parents' cellular genetics are passed on via the sperm and ovum, our resident probiotics are passed down from mother to child. This means two things: One, our probiotics recognize our cellular genetics as their permanent host environment.

Second, our cells and immune system recognize those strains of probiotics handed down by our mother as being residents. This intelligent co-recognition (or cognition) is not so special. After all, our immune system stores and recognizes the identities and characteristics of trillions of different microorganisms—remembering how to handle and defend against each and every one of them should they penetrate the body. Just as we can recognize millions of different faces—our immune system recognizes our probiotics, and our probiotics recognize our immune system.

This commingling and interactive cooperation between our immune system and our probiotics is precisely why our probiotic populations—and those supportive supplemental species—are so critically important to our body's health.

What supplemented probiotics do is set up an environment that stimulates our own strains to begin to re-grow. The supplemented strains produce lactic acid, nucleic acids and other nutrients that help establish this supportive environment.

What this all means is that we each have probiotic strains that are unique to us, and to some degree, are shared amongst our families. While we do inherit certain strains, the distinct combination and characteristics, together with subsequent genetic modification among those strains are unique. Just as no DNA and expression is exactly the same from person to person, no collection of probiotic colonies is the same from person to person. In other words, we each have our own special family of probiotic species and strains: Every host and family of probiotics is unique.

Probiotic Nourishment: Prebiotics

One of the most important factors in establishing a healthy environment for our probiotic colonies is making sure our probiotics have the right mix of nutrients. The foods our probiotic families favor are called prebiotics. In other words, some foods are particularly beneficial for probiotics. These are the oligosaccharides, fructooligosaccharides, galactooligosaccharides, and transgalactooligosaccharides. They are also referred to as inulin, FOS, GOS and TOS. Even 2.75 grams of one of these prebiotics will dramatically increase probiotic populations assuming resident colonies. Inulin, FOS, GOS and TOS are also antagonistic to toxic microorganism genera such as *Salmonella, Listeria, Campylobacter, Shigella* and *Vibrio*. These and other pathogenic bacteria tend to thrive from refined sugars and processed carbohydrates as opposed to the stacked saccharides like inulin, FOS, GOS and TOS.

Oligosaccharides are short stacks of simple yet mostly indigestible sugars (from the Greek *oligos*, meaning "few"). If the sugar molecule is fructose, the stacked molecule is called a fructooligosaccharide. If the sugar molecule is galactose, the stacked molecule is called a galactooligosaccharide. These molecules are very useful for our probiotics because they can be processed directly for energy as well as be combined with fatty acids to create cell wall structures and cellular communication combinations. This in turn helps probiotics colonize and multiply faster, and communicate better with the body's cells.

The oligosaccharides inulin and oligofructose are probably the most recognized prebiotics. Inulin is a naturally occurring carbohydrate used by plants for storage. It has been estimated that more than 36,000 plant species contain inulin in varying degrees (Carpita *et al.* 1989). The roots often contain the greatest amounts of inulin.

Commercial sources of inulin include Jerusalem artichoke, agave cactus and chicory. Chicory, the root of the Belgian endive, is known to contain some of the highest levels of both inulin at 15-20% and oligofructose at 5-10%. Inulin from agave has been described as highly branched. This gives it a higher solubility and digestibility than inulin derived from Jerusalem artichoke or chicory.

Prebiotic FOS-containing foods include garlic, leeks, bananas, fruits, soybeans, burdock root, asparagus, maple sugar, whole rye and whole wheat among others. Bananas contain one of the highest levels of FOS. This makes bananas a favorite food for both people and probiotics.

GOS and TOS are natural byproducts of milk. They are produced as lactose is enzymatically converted or hydrolyzed within the digestive tract. This process can also be done commercially. Before much of the recent research on prebiotics was performed, nutritionists simply thought of GOS and TOS as indigestible byproducts of milk.

Another element in plant foods providing probiotic nutrition for probiotics is the polyphenols. Polyphenols are groups of biochemicals produced in plants that include lignans, tannins, reservatrol, and flavonoids. There is some uncertainty as to which of these are most helpful to probiotic populations.

Some prebiotics have interesting side effects. For example, there seems to be a relationship between oligofructose inulin and calcium absorption. Inulin has been shown to improve calcium absorption by 20%, and yogurt supplemented with TOS can increase calcium absorption by 16% (van den Heuvel *et al.* 2000)

Galactooligosaccharides have another side effect that is important to note. Dr. Kari Shoaf and fellow researchers at the University of Nebraska (Shoaf *et al.* 2006) found in laboratory tests that galactooligosaccharides reduce the ability of *E. coli* to attach to human cells within tissue cultures. This effect was isolated from GOS' ability to nourish probiotics.

This all means that prebiotics provide more than nutrition to our probiotic colonies. These once-considered useless indigestible fibers provide an array of benefits not realized before. This of course illustrates the benefits of whole foods and whole dairy.

FOS and GOS have been known to cause digestive disturbance in rare cases. Such a digestive disturbance is likely caused by an absence of healthy probiotic colonies, however.

Conclusively, a preponderance of scientific literature indicates that probiotics thrive from a diet of plant-based natural foods with plenty of phytonutrients, while overly processed, sugary and meat diets tend to promote pathogenic bacteria and dangerous endotoxins. Let's discuss this latter point a bit further.

The Probiotic-Friendly Diet

Our health depends not just upon different populations of probiotics surviving within our bodies. They must also thrive and colonize to the greatest extent. This allows their colonies to be strong enough to counter invading pathogens. A weak probiotic colony is not much better than no colony at all, because weakened probiotic colonies are easily conquered in an invasion.

Even if some of probiotic colonies are supplemented, they will still be territorial, as the research has indicated. They will also be producing nutrients, helping us digest our foods. They will also help keep pathogenic bacteria populations at bay. As supplemented or transient strains grow, they also prepare our system for the regrowth of our resident strains.

It also appears evident there is a link between plant-based and dairy-based foods and probiotic colonization. While the below discussion is not intended as a thesis on any particular diet, the research below provides evidence for the association between plant-based and dairy-based foods and healthy probiotic colonization.

In 1980, Dr. Barry Goldin and fellow researchers reported a series of studies that connected diet and probiotics with a group of enzymes associated with the incidence of cancer. These enzymes were beta-glucuronidase, nitroreductase, azoreductase, and steroid 7-alpha-dehydroxylase.

Research on plant-based diets have shown lower levels of these enzymes. Apparently, these enzymes seem to have their origin from the presence of pathogenic bacteria in the intestines. In other words, these carcinogenic and pathogenic enzymes are actually endotoxins from pathogenic bacteria.

This led Dr. Goldin and associates to study the difference between these enzyme levels in omnivores and vegetarians. The researchers removed meat from the diets of a group of omnivores for 30 days. A significant reduction of steroid 7-alpha-dehydroxylase within the subjects resulted. With the addition of L. acidophilus supplementation, however, the vegetarian group also showed an increased reduction in beta-glucuronidase and nitroreductase.

Other studies have confirmed that various probiotic bacteria reduce levels of beta-glucuronidase. Beta-glucuronidase is one of the enzymes most associated with colon cancer. In Dr. Golden's research, thirty days after the withdrawal of the L. acidophilus supplementation, beta-glucuronidase enzymes returned to previous (prior to supplementation) levels.

Two years later Dr. Goldin and associates (Goldin et al. 1982) studied 10 vegetarian and 10 omnivore women. He found that the vegetarian women produced significantly lower levels of beta-glucuronidase than the omnivorous women—a result that was unrelated to any supplementation of probiotics.

The association between colon cancer and red meat diets has been shown conclusively in a variety of studies over the years. In an American Cancer Society (Chao et al. 2005) cohort study of 148,610 adults between the ages of 50 and 74 living in 21 states, higher intakes of red and processed meats were associated with rectal and colon cancer after other cancer variables were eliminated.

Other studies have confirmed the depletion of carcinogenic enzymes produced by pathogenic bacteria in vegetarian diets. Researchers from Finland's University of Kuopio (Ling and Hanninen 1992) tested 18 volunteers, who were randomly divided into either a control group (conventional animal products diet) or an extreme vegan diet for one month followed by a change back to their original diet. After only one week on the vegan diet, the researchers found that fecal urease levels decreased by 66%, cholylglycine hydrolase levels decreased by 55%, beta-glucuronidase levels decreased by 33%, and beta-glucosidase levels decreased by 40% in the vegan group, and continued through the month of consuming the vegan diet.

Serum levels of phenol and p-cresol—endotoxin byproducts of pathogenic bacteria—also significantly decreased in the vegan group. Within two weeks of returning to the animal diet, all of the pathogenic fecal enzyme levels returned to the levels before converting to the vegan diet. After one month of returning to the meat (omnivore) diet, the serum levels of toxins phenol and p-cresol returned to the levels before the change to the vegan diet. Meanwhile no changes in any of these enzyme or toxin levels occurred in the conventional (omnivore diet) control group.

A study published two years earlier by Huddinge University researchers (Johansson et al. 1990) also confirmed the same results. The conversion of an omnivore diet to a lacto-vegetarian diet significantly reduced levels of beta-glucuronidase, beta-glucosidase, and sulphatase from fecal samples.

A further connection between plant-based foods, pathogenic bacterial enzymes and cancer was confirmed by another study conducted at Sweden's Huddinge University and University Hospital (Johansson et al. 1998) almost a decade later. Dr. Johansson and associates measured the effect of switching from an omnivore diet to a lacto-vegetarian diet and back to an omnivore diet with regard to mutagenicity—an environment rich with pathogenic bacteria and the tendency for tumor formation. Twenty non-smoking and normal weight volunteers switched to a lacto-vegetarian diet for one year. Their feces were examined for mutagenicity (using mutagenic and pathogenic bacteria) at the start of the study, at three months, at six months and at twelve months after beginning the vegetarian diet. Then they tested the subjects at three years after converting back to an omnivore diet. Following the switch to the lacto-vegetarian diet, all mutagenic parameters significantly decreased among the urine and feces of the subjects.

The clear conclusion we must take away from this research is that probiotics prefer plant-based foods, and plant-based foods stimulate the colonization of probiotics, which inhibit the growth of pathogenic bacteria and cancer. Since the levels of beta-glucuronidase fall significantly following the addition of probiotics when more plant foods are added, we can correlate that probiotics must be removing and controlling the pathogenic bacteria that produce these enzymes. Because beta-glucuronidase levels are higher in a plant-poor diet, we can conclude that eating meat discourages the growth of probiotics and encourages the growth of pathogenic bacteria that produce beta-glucuronidase. We can also then conclude that since vegetarians (immediately and to a greater extent after probiotic supplementation) produce lower levels of beta-glucuronidase, plant-abundant diets also promote the growth of probiotics and decrease the risk of colon cancer.

A contributing mechanism of this effect was found in Dr. Goldin's 1982 research, and confirmed the usefulness of plant and dairy foods in our diet. Plant-based foods also tend to move through the digestive tract faster. A slower-moving digestive tract allows for more time for pathogenic bacteria to colonize. Diets without a good supply of plant-based foods invite increased populations of pathogenic bacteria.

The reader might wonder what this has to do with oral probiotics. Everything. Oral probiotics are cooperative bacteria. They thrive in a positive-growth medium with the right pH. The medium created in our intestines from our foods is typically mirrored in our oral cavities with respect to pH.

Consider dairy foods. One of the most nutritious prebiotics for most probiotics is contained in dairy. Probiotic bacteria love to ferment within dairy environments. This is why they readily live within cow's milk, colostrum and human breast milk. They are comfortable within the pH of milk. They also utilize milk's lactose and the GOS that comes from dairy for food. This is why milk curdles so fast. Probiotics quickly expand their colonies within whole milk. They love this environment..

Probiotic Hydration

Our probiotics need water just as we do. Our mucous membranes all require sufficient water for secreting mucus and providing an environment attractive to probiotics. Like most other organisms, the body of a probiotic is mostly water. Water thus serves as a critical nutrient for our microflora friends. Probiotics also require a wet environment to maintain their movement, communications and colonization processes. We should also remember that prebiotics are fibrous, and thus require water to move them through the digestive tract.

The question is how much water is necessary? Conventional advice has suggested around six to eight 8-oz glasses per day for an adult. In 2004, the National Academy of Sciences released a study indicating that the average woman requires approximately 91 ounces of water per day, while men meet their needs with about 125 ounces per day. This study also indicated that approximately 80% of this comes from drinking water and beverages, and 20% comes from food. Therefore, we can assume a minimum of 73 ounces of fresh water/beverages for the average adult woman and 100 ounces of fresh water/beverages for the average adult man should cover our minimum needs. That is significantly more water than the standard eight glasses per day (64 ounces)—especially for men. It is not surprising that some health professionals have suggested that 50-75% of Americans suffer from chronic dehydration. Dr. Batmanghelidj, one of the world's most respected researchers on human hydration, suggests 1/2 ounce of water per pound of body weight. Additional water should be consumed before and after strenuous activity. Extremes in temperature and elevation increase our water requirements as well. Additional water is also required during periods of fever or increased sweating.

Hydration experts agree that as soon as we feel thirsty, our bodies are already experiencing dehydration. Becoming consciously thirsty is the point where cellular and probiotic damage is occurring. Our thirst sensation decreases as we age, so it is much easier to become dehydrated in our later years. Natural mineralized water is critical for the smooth running of all of our cells and probiotics. Tissue systems likely to suffer first during dehydration include our mucous membranes, digestive tract, joints, eyes and liver. Some health experts have estimated as little as a 5% loss of body water will decrease physical performance by up to 30%. Watching our urine to make sure we are getting enough water is a good idea. Our urine color should range from light yellow to clear. Darker urine indicates a state of dehydration.

Probiotic Foods

Probiotic foods can contribute to healthy probiotic colonies among the mouth, pharynx and nasal cavity. This is accomplished simply because as we eat these foods some will stay back and begin to set up shop, at least temporarily. As they do this, they attack pathogenic colonies and stimulate growth of our resident probiotic strains by contributing to a culture-positive environment. Here are a few probiotic foods to consider adding to the diet:

Yogurt: Typically produced with *L. bulgaricus, S. thermophilus* and sometimes *L. acidophilus.* Pasteurization kills probiotic colonies so pasteurized yogurt is not helpful unless supplemental strains have been added after pasteurization. Note that *L. acidophilus* yogurt colonies will likely be overwhelmed by *L. bulgaricus* in yogurt blends that use *L. acidophilus.*

Kefir: A traditional drink of Eastern Europe and southern Russia, Georgia, Armenia and Azerbaijan. Kefir grains with active cultured probiotics are mixed with milk to produce this fermented beverage.

Buttermilk: A soured milk beverage curdled from cream traditionally using probiotic bacteria for curdling. Today, forced curdling is done using acidic products like lemon, vinegar or tartar, so not all commercial buttermilks have probiotics. This also goes for cottage cheese and butter. All were traditional probiotic foods, curdled with natural probiotics derived from cow's milk. Again, commercial versions are typically produced with lactic acid or other acids.

Kim Chi: A fermented cabbage made with ginger, garlic, red pepper, green onions, oil and other ingredients. *Lactobacillus kimchii* and *L. plantarum* are typical probiotics cultured in kim chi.

Miso: Miso is an ancient food from Japan. Traditional miso can contain more than 160 strains of probiotic bacteria. Miso is fermented from beans and grains. The original fungi spore is called koji, or *Aspergillus oryzae.*

Shoyu: This traditional form of soy sauce is made with cooked soybeans, wheat and again koji, or *Aspergillus oryzae.* The aging process for shoyu depends upon storage temperature and cooking methods used.

Tempeh: This is an aged and fermented soybean food containing a combination of probiotics. Tempeh starter often contains *Rhyzopus oryzae, Rhizopus oligosporus* or both. Other probiotics arise with the fermentation.

Kombucha Tea: This is an ancient fermented beverage from the orient. Its use dates back many centuries, to China and Taiwanese royalty. Kombucha was eventually popularized in Russia and Eastern Europe. Kombucha tea can contain a number of probiotics, including *Acetobacter xylinum, Acetobacter xylinoides, Glucobacter gluconicum, Acetobacter aceti, Saccharomycodes ludwigii, Schizo-*

saccharomyces pombe, and *Picha fermentans*—and other fungi from the *Schizosaromyces* genus.

Lassi: A traditional and popular beverage from India. It is a blend of liquefied yogurt with fruit pulp—often mango is used in the traditional form of lassi.

Sauerkraut: A traditional German fermented food. Sauerkraut is made by blending shredded cabbage and pickling salts into a fermentation culture not unlike kimchi.

Probiotic Oral Hygiene

There has been significant research on dental decay, plaque and gingivitis over the decades. Most of this research has focused upon removing plaque and removing the bacteria that generate plaque. The logic is that the acids within plaque have been associated with dental decay. The acidic content within plaque eats away at the enamel lining in the teeth, and eventually carves holes into the dentin of the teeth.

As a result, it has made good sense to remove the plaque from the teeth through flossing and brushing after meals and upon waking. This has also been proven by the research: Those who brush after meals and floss regularly tend to have less dental decay.

The problem we get into is that even with good brushing habits and regular flossing, there is still an epidemic of periodontal disease and gingivitis among the world's population—especially among those from wealthier countries where dental hygiene is most available. What is it about these societies—even among those who brush well—that still allows for this epidemic of gum disease?

Problems with Gum Disease

We might wonder why gum disease is such an important topic to discuss. The fact is, gum disease—which includes periodontal disease and gingivitis—has been linked to a number of disorders.

An advanced case of periodontal disease, for example, opens up the spaces between the gums and the teeth. This gum-teeth attachment is critical for keeping infection levels down within the roots of the teeth. Once "pockets" form, pathogenic bacteria can harbor within, and grow in colony size. As this takes place, their production of acids can eat away at the roots of the teeth, rotting out the teeth and infecting the jawbone.

An infection of the jawbone can create a number of problems. Once bacteria begin to grow within the jawbone, they can destroy the jaw and the surrounding tissues. This can lead to further complications.

Worse, bacteria that are housed within these pockets (and/or their endotoxins) can escape into the bloodstream. As this occurs, they can damage tissues, blood vessels and even the heart. Research has confirmed these suspicions. Research has identified that periodontal disease sufferers have a significantly higher risk of coronary artery disease compared to those without periodontal disease.

Still, there have been doubters, as the mechanisms are not fully understood. To settle some of the doubt, researchers from the Veterans Affairs Medical Center and the Oregon Evidence-based Practice Center reviewed the results of seven relevant studies that studied the link between periodontal disease and coronary heart disease. They found that periodontal disease sufferers had a 1.24 to 1.34 higher relative risk for coronary heart disease (Humphrey *et al.* 2008) than those without periodontal disease.

Other studies, such as a recent study of 17,802 men and women (Ridker and Silvertown 2008) have shown that periodontal disease may spark increases in inflammatory responses that can translate to atherosclerosis and atherothrombosis. This converts to a higher risk of stroke and other cardiovascular disorders.

Researchers from the Department of Periodontics at the University of Texas Health Science Center (Mealey and Rose 2008) looked at a broader range of associations between inflammatory diseases and periodontal disease. They established that, *"Periodontal inflammation is associated with an elevated systemic inflammatory state and an increased risk of major cardiovascular events such as myocardial infarction and stroke, adverse pregnancy outcomes such as preeclampsia, low birth weight, and preterm birth, and altered glycemic control in people with diabetes."*

This inclusion of issues such as pregnancy problems and diabetes 'seals the deal' on the importance of keeping our oral bacteria balanced.

How to Reduce Our Risk of Periodontal Disease

How can we avoid or reverse periodontal disease? Certainly, the research supports brushing after meals and after waking. Flossing and oral irrigation (for example, the Waterpik®) are also extremely effective at reducing plaque and dental decay.

A study from the University of Nebraska's Medical College (Barnes *et al.* 2005) found that water irrigation was more effective than flossing after fourteen days, and just as effective as flossing at 28 days for removing plaque, reducing gum bleeding, and preventing gingivitis infections. Both flossing and water irrigation are better.

Annual or semi-annual cleanings are critical. We can also learn techniques for removing plaque with flossing, water irrigation and brushing from our dental hygienist during these cleanings.

However, the use of chemical toothpastes and mouthwashes to lower infection is another topic altogether. Yes, research has indeed confirmed that chemical antimicrobial mouthwashes and toothpastes (also called dentifrices) will lower total coliform and plate counts in the mouth. They will certainly lower bacteria counts immediately following their use.

What happens afterwards, however? Once the antimicrobial chemicals reside, oral cavity bacteria once again recolonize the oral cavity and associated cavities. What species of bacteria will arise at this point? Will they be our resident probiotic colonies, or perhaps the pathogenic colonies that cause periodontal disease?

While the research is mostly silent on the specific types of bacteria that arise following antimicrobial mouthwashes and dentifrices, we can logically deduce the result from research showing that pathogenic bacteria tend to grow faster in the absence of oral probiotics. The risk of fast regrowth is increased by eating refined foods and refined sweeteners.

In order to keep pathogenic bacteria populations low using antiseptics, they must be used on a constant basis. Antiseptic rinses and mouthwashes must be used multiple times daily to maintain their effects. Shortly after use, pathogenic bacteria will regrow in colony strength, possibly even surpassing original levels over time.

We see this same effect among intestinal bacteria and the use of antibiotics. Several studies have illustrated that aggressive pathogenic microorganisms expand the fastest after a course of antibiotics in the absence of probiotic supplementation. This yields a higher risk of re-infection or co-infection with other fast-growing microorganisms, with a combined effect of a reduction in probiotic colonies. Antibiotics have a similar effect as antiseptic mouthwashes.

Supplementing with oral probiotics will reduce pathogenic bacteria counts by increasing probiotic colonies. Oral probiotic supplementation thus reduces periodontal disease and dental caries risk.

The bottom line is that when both probiotic bacteria and pathogenic bacteria are knocked out, pathogenic bacteria become more aggressive immediately thereafter. Their populations are more prevalent among our surroundings. Probiotics are more exclusive within organisms such as humans and other animals. The more opportunistic pathogenic organisms that have become resistant to the stressors of temperature and relative acidity are more readily available within our immediate environment. They will thus expand more quickly in an uncontrolled environment.

Probiotics, on the other hand, can grow aggressively, but they require a particular type of acidic medium and a particular type of food source, notably FOS, GOS and TOS, as discussed earlier. Pathogenic bacteria, on the other hand, will thrive from nearly any sort of simple sugar molecule or carbohydrate. For this reason, they will grow quickly amongst a diet of processed starches and sugars. This of course is the connection between dental caries and diet. Sugar and processed carbs promote the growth of pathogenic bacteria that metabolize these sugars to produce endotoxins, which include acid-forming plaque.

Over the last few centuries, many traditional health proponents have suggested that a diet of simple sugary foods results in an acidic environment, creating a greater propensity for infection. Conventional medical science argues with this assumption from a purely biochemical stance, not understanding how sugar is utilized by pathogenic bacteria. Now that we see how pathogenic bacteria thrive from refined sugar and produce a variety of acids, we now can understand the relationship between sugar, acids and disease.

The Healthy Oral Regimen

Brushing in the morning and after meals is a good place to start. Brushing with a soft bristle brush or sonic brush will stimulate circulation within the gums and help clear pathogens.

The question becomes; what kind of dentifrice or toothpaste should we use? There are a few brands of natural toothpaste available today. These use a minimum of chemicals that can damage our oral probiotics, yet contain good cleaning agents.

In the absence of these, diluted baking soda can alkalize and neutralize acids on and around teeth. However, brushing with baking soda can also remove enamel. Brush first, and then dilute a teaspoon of soda in a glass of water and swish it around the mouth and through the teeth before spitting out. Some natural toothpastes use baking soda with anti-abrasives, so these can work.

In addition to brushing; *flossing, gargling, swishing* and *water irrigation* (e.g., Waterpik®) are critical. A new machine called Airfloss® combines air with water droplets. All these strategies help reduce pathogenic bacteria counts and endotoxins in the mouth. *Liquid chlorophyll*—praised by holistic doctors for stimulating healthy gums—can also useful as a rinse and or irrigation additive.

In addition, the Ayurvedic practice of *oil pulling* has been shown to reduce pathogenic oral bacteria (Asokan et al. 2011). To oil-pull, simply lightly swish (don't gargle or swallow) a teaspoon of virgin sesame seed oil or coconut oil between the teeth and gums.

A *tongue cleaner* is also useful for decreasing oral pathogens.

Most of us who have visited with a dental hygienist know how to brush properly. While brushing the enamel is certainly important and should not be overlooked, brushing too harshly and in the wrong direction can harm the gums over time. Best to keep a more circular motion over the enamel and lightly massage the gums.

Our *gums* require more care than do our teeth. The gums provide the foundation for healthy root systems. Healthy gums deliver nutrients, blood, oxygen and immune cells to our teeth; helping the dental pulp, dentin, roots, and enamel remain strong and better able to prevent infection within.

When the gums are beat up by harsh brushing and flossing, they will recede over time. As they recede, the roots and nerves become exposed to the environment of the mouth, which includes pathogenic bacteria and their acids, which will eat away into the roots, tooth enamel and dentin. This can cause a severe type of decay, which requires serious dental repair.

Receding gums also produce more *pockets* between the teeth and the gums. Aggressive bacteria we described in Chapter Five will set up shop in these pockets, and grow to outrageous colony sizes. They will produce acids and endotoxins such as leukotoxin, which can leak into the bloodstream. One in the bloodstream, these *toxins* will damage arteries and tissues. There is also evidence of some of these bacteria translocating around the body through the bloodstream.

While they are sometimes necessary to repair damage from tooth decay, *root canals* should be avoided if there is any alternative offered by the dentist. This is because root canal surgery kills the tooth by removing the nerves and blood supply to the nerve root. This prevents the body from defending this region.

This lack of innervation and circulation combined with the possibility of future cracking opens us up to an infection of the dead root canals. Often the bacteria that end up infecting a dead root canal are spirochetes, which, as we described earlier, can be extremely dangerous when they set up shop.

Along with this oral regimen, we can focus upon stimulating *the regrowth of our resident oral probiotic colonies.* The foundation for this is a *healthy lifestyle with exercise; a whole-food diet with plenty of fiber and few refined foods; sufficient drinking water;* and the right mix of *oral probiotic supplements.*

The most efficient way to stimulate our probiotic colonies is with the supplementation of strains such as *Lactobacillus salivarius, Lactobacillus reuteri,* and *Streptococcus salivarius.* We can choose *lozenges* or *gums* to accomplish this, but lozenges are probably the most effective because of their timed release.

We can also support our oral probiotics with *probiotic foods* and *intestinal probiotic supplements.* They will contribute to an overall positive probiotic environment throughout the body, lending to the right fermentation medium within which to grow.

Feeding our resident oral colonies is critical. This means plenty of *fresh vegetables, fruits, root foods, grains* and *beans*, along with *fermented dairy* and *other cultured foods*—including foods like vinegar, sauerkraut and yogurt. This kind of diet will supply our probiotics with nourishment and a good pH environment for colony growth.

Careful and limited use of antimicrobial chemicals taken into the mouth—such as those in many *antiseptic mouthwashes and toothpastes*—will also give our probiotic colonies the ability to remain in control of our oral cavity, nasal cavity and pharynx with little resistance. If we use an antiseptic occasionally, we can follow this with an increase in oral probiotic supplementation.

A variety of manufactured chemicals added to many foods such as *preservatives* and *food colorings* also hamper the growth of probiotic populations. Preservatives, remember, are added to foods to specifically deter bacterial growth and eliminate food spoilage. The problem with this strategy is that foods containing preservatives will also retard our own probiotic bacteria populations.

Without a balanced *whole-food diet* with plenty of plant-based *fiber*, we will effectively starve or under-nourish our probiotic populations. Foods lacking in fiber, high in *trans-fats*, high in *refined sugar* and/or *low in nutrient content* discourage probiotic growth and encourage pathogenic populations. Diets high in *fried foods* and *saturated animal fats* have been shown to decrease healthy flora. This is due to the release of anti-probiotic enzymes like beta-glucuronidase, nitroreductase, azoreductase, and steroid 7-alpha-dehydroxylase. These enzymes had been linked with colon cancer as well as probiotic declines.

Medications such as oral contraceptives, NSAIDS, corticosteroids, and other chemical pharmaceuticals can kill off or dramatically shrink oral probiotic populations. Following this die off, pathogenic bacteria arise in stronger colonies. For this reason, oral probiotic supplementation can be alternated with any medication use. In addition, after any the medication course, probiotic dosages can be increased for a few weeks to help rebuild lost colonies.

There are three ancient Ayurvedic oral hygiene practices applicable to oral health. The first is *drinking a room-temperature glass of water before eating* in the morning. This, according to the ancient tradition, allows our saliva and mucopolysaccharides built up in our mouth over the night to be flushed down to the lower esophagus and stomach. This contributes to the health of the mucosal membranes of our throat and esophagus. The mechanics of this are now better understood in light of the fact that our oral cavity probiotic colonies will strengthen overnight. Washing them down in the morning allows our upper digestive tract to be inoculated with probiotic colonies together with their fermentation culture.

Another Ayurvedic practice is the *nasal lavage*. Here, warm water (a pinch of natural salt with a pinch of baking soda can help) is poured between the nostrils on each side with our head turned to the side. This can cleanse the nasal cavities and flush pathogenic colonies. A neutral salt/baking soda mixture can add an alkalizing effect, which will deter pathogenic bacteria growth and stimulate probiotic growth.

Tongue cleaning is also a traditional practice introduced by Ayurveda. Tongue cleaning utilizes a metal (preferable to plastic) tongue scraping tool to reach back onto the back of the tongue and lightly "scrape" or pull forward, out of the mouth, the film of bacteria that resides on the surface of the tongue. Because pathogenic bacteria often inhabit the back of the tongue, this can significantly reduce their populations.

Probiotic Night Owls

Our probiotics shift into high gear when our bodies are sleeping. As we sleep, probiotics come into full bloom and work to manage their local environments. This means that probiotics go into battle mode against pathogenic microorganisms when we sleep. They also stimulate the production of particular types of T-cells, B-cells and various cytokines. This is accomplished through the pro-

ORAL PROBIOTICS

duction of various chemical signals such as prolactin put out by probiotics.

If we are sleeping poorly and stressed during our daylight hours, our probiotic populations are probably also stressed, and weakened. For this reason, supplemental probiotics in therapeutic doses can assist in maintaining a healthy environment for probiotic growth. They can also help protect the body from pathogenic bacteria growth during a time when our resident populations are minimized.

A great way to accomplish this is by taking oral probiotic lozenges prior to falling asleep. As we drift off, supplemented probiotic colonies go to work to manage the bad guys while creating an environment useful for the regrowth of our resident strains. By morning we should have significant colonization of the oral cavity.

In Conclusion

Probiotics are conscious organisms. They are unique living creatures, worth our respect and appreciation. They are also our partners in the health of our body. Certainly, bacteria may not be as aware and conscious of the larger physical world as we might. Still, we know they are aware, because laboratory studies show that they react and adapt to threats to their surroundings. These studies also show they vigorously defend their territories.

By protecting and supporting our probiotic colonies with a healthy diet, supplementation and a reduction of antiseptic chemicals, we can maintain a balance of living organisms within our body. This living balance is dependent upon healthy oral probiotic colonies. Healthy oral bacteria can help us achieve a level of protection that many modern antimicrobial strategies cannot provide in the long run. Our probiotic colonies can prevent disease and stimulate our immune system in its processes of wound repair and detoxification. They can also help reduce the endotoxins that pathogenic bacteria leave behind to poison our bodies.

We owe it to our bodies to try to reach a healthy balance among our oral bacteria. This means we have to support them. We must learn what helps them survive, and adapt our activities to promote their survival. As we learn to cooperate and work with our probiotics, they will stimulate the health of our bodies. What a deal!

Science will soon discover that the rates of infection, epidemics and pandemics relate directly to the strength and health of our oral probiotic colonies. Our oral probiotics are the gatekeepers for our body because they guard the largest entryways into the body: Our mouth and sinuses. In other words, when our oral probiotics are healthy and balanced, our bodies will stay healthier.

As the boxing champion Jack Dempsey once said, *"The best defense is a good offense."* It only makes sense to put our body's best offensive health team on the field: Our oral probiotics.

References and Bibliography

Aas JA, Paster BJ, Stokes LN, Olsen I, Dewhirst FE. Defining the normal bacterial flora of the oral cavity. *J Clin Microbiol.* 2005 Nov;43(11):5721-32.

Adoga AS, Otene AA, Yiltok SJ, Adekwu A, Nwaorgu OG. Cervical necrotizing fasciitis: case series and review of literature. *Niger J Med.* 2009 Apr-Jun;18(2):203-7.

Agarwal KN, Bhasin SK, Faridi MM, Mathur M, Gupta S. *Lactobacillus casei* in the control of acute diarrhea—a pilot study. *Indian Pediatr.* 2001 Aug;38(8):905-10.

Agerholm-Larsen L, Raben A, Haulrik N, Hansen AS, Manders M, Astrup A. Effect of 8 week intake of probiotic milk products on risk factors for cardiovascular diseases. *Eur J Clin Nutr.* 2000 Apr;54(4):288-97.

Agustina R, Lukito W, Firmansyah A, Suhardjo HN, Murniati D, Bindels J. The effect of early nutritional supplementation with a mixture of probiotic, prebiotic, fiber and micronutrients in infants with acute diarrhea in Indonesia. *Asia Pac J Clin Nutr.* 2007;16(3):435-42.

Ahmed M, Prasad J, Gill H, Stevenson L, Gopal P. Impact of consumption of different levels of *Bifidobacterium lactis* HN019 on the intestinal microflora of elderly human subjects. *J Nutr Health Aging.* 2007 Jan-Feb;11(1):26-31.

Ahmed, AA, McCarthy RD, Porter GA. Effect of of milk constituents on hepatic cholesterogenesis. *Atherosclerosis.* 1979;32:347-57.

Ahola AJ, Yli-Knuuttila H, Suomalainen T, Poussa T, Ahlström A, Meurman JH, Korpela R. Short-term consumption of probiotic-containing cheese and its effect on dental caries risk factors. *Arch Oral Biol.* 2002 Nov;47(11):799-804.

Aihara K, Kajimoto O, Hirata H, Takahashi R, Nakamura Y. Effect of powdered fermented milk with *Lactobacillus helveticus* on subjects with high-normal blood pressure or mild hypertension. *J Am Coll Nutr.* 2005 Aug;24(4):257-65.

Akil I, Yilmaz O, Kurutepe S, Degerli K, Kavukcu S. Influence of oral intake of *Saccharomyces boulardii* on *Escherichia coli* in enteric flora. *Pediatr Nephrol.* 2006 Jun;21(6):807-10.

Allaker RP, Douglas CW. Novel anti-microbial therapies for dental plaque-related diseases. *Int J Antimicrob Agents.* 2009 Jan;33(1):8-13.

Allen SJ, Okoko B, Martinez E, Gregorio G, Dans LF. Probiotics for treating infectious diarrhea. *The Cochrane Library.* 2004;3. Chichester, UK: John Wiley & Sons, Ltd.

Amenta M, Cascio MT, Di Fiore P, Venturini I. Diet and chronic constipation. Benefits of oral supplementation with symbiotic zir fos (*Bifidobacterium longum* W11 + FOS Actilight). *Acta Biomed.* 2006 Dec;77(3):157-62.

Anderson JW, Gilliland SE. Effect of fermented milk (yogurt) containing *Lactobacillus acidophilus* L1 on serum cholesterol in hypercholesterolemic humans. *J Am Coll Nutr.* 1999 Feb;18(1):43-50.

Anukam K, Osazuwa E, Ahonkhai I, Ngwu M, Osemene G, Bruce AW, Reid G. Augmentation of antimicrobial metronidazole therapy of bacterial vaginosis with oral probiotic *Lactobacillus rhamnosus* GR-1 and *Lactobacillus reuteri* RC-14: randomized, double-blind, placebo controlled trial. *Microbes Infect.* 2006 May;8(6):1450-4.

Anukam KC, Osazuwa E, Osemene GI, Ehigiagbe F, Bruce AW, Reid G. Clinical study comparing probiotic *Lactobacillus* GR-1 and RC-14 with metronidazole vaginal gel to treat symptomatic bacterial vaginosis. *Microbes Infect.* 2006 Oct;8(12-13):2772-6.

Anukam KC, Osazuwa EO, Osadolor HB, Bruce AW, Reid G. Yogurt containing probiotic *Lactobacillus rhamnosus* GR-1 and *L. reuteri* RC-14 helps resolve moderate diarrhea and increases CD4 count in HIV/AIDS patients. *J Clin Gastroenterol.* 2008 Mar;42(3):239-43.

Araki K, Shinozaki T, Irie Y, Miyazawa Y. Trial of oral administration of *Bifidobacterium breve* for the prevention of rotavirus infections. *Kansenshogaku Zasshi.* 1999 Apr;73(4):305-10.

Armstrong BK. Absorption of vitamin B12 from the human colon. *Am J Clin Nutr.* 1968;21:298-9.

Armuzzi A, Cremonini F, Bartolozzi F, Canducci F, Candelli M, Ojetti V, Cammarota G, Anti M, De Lorenzo A, Pola P, Gasbarrini G, Gasbarrini A. The effect of oral administration of *Lactobacillus* GG on antibiotic-associated gastrointestinal side-effects during *Helicobacter pylori* eradication therapy. *Aliment Pharmacol Ther.* 2001 Feb;15(2):163-9.

Arrigo G, D'Angelo A. Achromycin and anaphylactic shock. *Riv Patol Clin.* 1959 Oct;14:719-22.

Arunachalam K, Gill HS, Chandra RK. Enhancement of natural immune function by dietary consumption of *Bifidobacterium lactis* (HN019). *Eur J Clin Nutr.* 2000 Mar;54(3):263-7.

Arvola T, Laiho K, Torkkeli S, Mykkänen H, Salminen S, Maunula L, Isolauri E. Prophylactic *Lactobacillus* GG reduces antibiotic-associated diarrhea in children with respiratory infections: a randomized study. *Pediatrics.* 1999 Nov;104(5):e64.

Aso Y, Akaza H, Kotake T, Tsukamoto T, Imai K, Naito S. Preventive effect of a *Lactobacillus casei* preparation on the recurrence of superficial bladder cancer in a double-blind trial. The BLP Study Group. *Eur Urol.* 1995;27(2):104-9.

Aso Y, Akazan H. Prophylactic effect of a *Lactobacillus casei* preparation on the recurrence of superficial bladder cancer. *BLP Study Group. Urol Int.* 1992;49(3):125-9.

Asokan S, Kumar RS, Emmadi P, Raghuraman R, Sivakumar N. Effect of oil pulling on halitosis and micro-organisms causing halitosis: a randomized controlled pilot trial. J Indian Soc Pedod Prev Dent. 2011 Apr-Jun;29(2):90-4.

Ataie-Jafari A, Larijani B, Alavi Majd H, Tahbaz F. Cholesterol-lowering effect of probiotic yogurt in comparison with ordinary yogurt in mildly to moderately hypercholesterolemic subjects. *Ann Nutr Metab.* 2009;54(1):22-7.

Backster C. *Primary Perception: Biocommunication with Plants, Living Foods, and Human Cells.* Anza, CA: White Rose Millennium Press, 2003.

Bai AP, Ouyang Q, Xiao XR, Li SF. Probiotics modulate inflammatory cytokine secretion from inflamed mucosa in active ulcerative colitis. *Int J Clin Pract.* 2006 Mar;60(3):284-8.

Baik HW. Nutritional therapy in gastrointestinal disease. *Korean J Gastroenterol.* 2004 Jun;43(6):331-40.

Baker SM. *Detoxification and Healing.* Chicago: Contemporary Books, 2004.

Balimane P, Yong-Haen H, Chong S. Current Industrial Practices of Assessing Permeability and P-Glycoprotein Interaction. *J AAPS* 2006; 8(1).

Ballentine R. *Diet & Nutrition: A holistic approach.* Honesdale, PA: Himalayan Int., 1978.

Ballentine RM. *Radical Healing.* New York: Harmony Books, 1999.

Balli F, Bertolani P, Giberti G, Amarri S. High-dose oral bacteria-therapy for chronic non-specific diarrhea of infancy. *Pediatr Med Chir.* 1992 Jan-Feb;14(1):13-5.

Barnes CM, Russell CM, Reinhardt RA, Payne JB, Lyle DM. Comparison of irrigation to floss as an adjunct to tooth brushing: effect on bleeding, gingivitis, and supragingival plaque. *J Clin Dent.* 2005;16(3):71-7.

Baron M. A patented strain of Bacillus coagulans increased immune response to viral challenge. *Postgrad Med.* 2009 Mar;121(2):114-8.

Bartram HP, Scheppach W, Gerlach S, Ruckdeschel G, Kelber E, Kasper H. Does yogurt enriched with *Bifidobacterium longum* affect colonic microbiology and fecal metabolites in health subjects? *Am J Clin Nutr.* 1994 Feb;59(2):428-32.

Basu S, Chatterjee M, Ganguly S, Chandra PK. Effect of *Lactobacillus rhamnosus* GG in persistent diarrhea in Indian children: a randomized controlled trial. *J Clin Gastroenterol.* 2007 Sep;41(8):756-60.

Basu S, Chatterjee M, Ganguly S, Chandra PK. Efficacy of *Lactobacillus rhamnosus* GG in acute watery diarrhoea of Indian children: a randomised controlled trial. *J Paediatr Child Health.* 2007 Dec;43(12):837-42.

Batmanghelidj F. *Your Body's Many Cries for Water.* 2nd Ed. Vienna, VA: Global Health, 1997.

Beausoleil M, Fortier N, Guénette S, L'ecuyer A, Savoie M, Franco M, Lachaine J, Weiss K. Effect of a fermented milk combining *Lactobacillus acidophilus* Cl1285 and *Lactobacillus casei* in the prevention of antibiotic-associated diarrhea: a randomized, double-blind, placebo-controlled trial. *Can J Gastroenterol.* 2007 Nov;21(11):732-6.

Bengmark S. Immunonutrition: role of biosurfactants, fiber, and probiotic bacteria. *Nutrition.* 1998 Jul-Aug;14(7-8):585-94.

Billoo AG, Memon MA, Khaskheli SA, Murtaza G, Iqbal K, Saeed Shekhani M, Siddiqi AQ. Role of a probiotic (*Saccharomyces boulardii*) in management and prevention of diarrhoea. *World J Gastroenterol.* 2006 Jul 28;12(28):4557-60.

Bin-Nun A, Bromiker R, Wilschanski M, Kaplan M, Rudensky B, Caplan M, Hammerman C. Oral probiotics prevent necrotizing enterocolitis in very low birth weight neonates. *J Pediatr.* 2005 Aug;147(2):192-6.

Bliakher MS, Fedorova IM, Lopatina TK, Arkhipov SN, Kapustin IV, Ramazanova ZK, Karpova NV, Ivanov VA, Sharapov NV. Acilact and improvement of the health status of sickly children. *Vestn Ross Akad Med Nauk.* 2005;(12):32-5.

Bode C, Bode JC. Effect of alcohol consumption on the gut. *Best Pract Res Clin Gastroenterol.* 2003 Aug;17(4):575-92.

Boivin DB, Czeisler CA. Resetting of circadian melatonin and cortisol rhythms in humans by ordinary room light. *Neuroreport.* 1998 Mar 30;9(5):779-82.

Boivin DB, Duffy JF, Kronauer RE, Czeisler CA. Dose-response relationships for resetting of human circadian clock by light. *Nature.* 1996 Feb 8;379(6565):540-2.

Bongaerts GP, Severijnen RS. Preventive and curative effects of probiotics in atopic patients. *Med Hypotheses.* 2005;64(6):1089-92.

Böttcher MF, Abrahamsson TR, Fredriksson M, Jakobsson T, Björkstén B. Low breast milk TGF-beta2 is induced by *Lactobacillus reuteri* supplementation and associates with reduced risk of sensitization during infancy. *Pediatr Allergy Immunol.* 2008 Sep;19(6):497-504.

Boylan R, Li Y, Simeonova L, Sherwin G, Kreismann J, Craig RG, Ship JA, McCutcheon JA. Reduction in bacterial contamination of toothbrushes using the Violight ultraviolet light activated toothbrush sanitizer. *Am J Dent.* 2008 Oct;21(5):313-7.

REFERENCES AND BIBLIOGRAPHY

Brasseur JG, Nicosia MA, Pal A, Miller LS. Function of longitudinal vs circular muscle fibers in esophageal peristalsis, deduced with mathematical modeling. *World J Gastroenterol.* 2007 Mar 7;13(9):1335-46.

Bu LN, Chang MH, Ni YH, Chen HL, Cheng CC. *Lactobacillus casei* rhamnosus Lcr35 in children with chronic constipation. *Pediatr Int.* 2007 Aug;49(4):485-90.

Burton JP, Chilcott CN, Moore CJ, Speiser G, Tagg JR. A preliminary study of the effect of probiotic Streptococcus salivarius K12 on oral malodour parameters. *J Appl Microbiol.* 2006 Apr;100(4):754-64.

Burton JP, Chilcott CN, Tagg JR. The rationale and potential for the reduction of oral malodour using Streptococcus salivarius probiotics. *Oral Dis.* 2005;11 Suppl 1:29-31.

Burton JP, Wescombe PA, Moore CJ, Chilcott CN, Tagg JR. Safety assessment of the oral cavity probiotic Streptococcus salivarius K12. *Appl Environ Microbiol.* 2006 Apr;72(4):3050-3.

Caglar E, Kavaloglu SC, Kuscu OO, Sandalli N, Holgerson PL, Twetman S. Effect of chewing gums containing xylitol or probiotic bacteria on salivary mutans streptococci and lactobacilli. *Clin Oral Investig.* 2007 Dec;11(4):425-9.

Caglar E, Kuscu OO, Cildir SK, Kuvvetli SS, Sandalli N. A probiotic lozenge administered medical device and its effect on salivary mutans streptococci and lactobacilli. *Int J Paediatr Dent.* 2008 Jan;18(1):35-9.

Caglar E, Kuscu OO, Selvi Kuvvetli S, Kavaloglu Cildir S, Sandalli N, Twetman S. Short-term effect of ice-cream containing *Bifidobacterium lactis* Bb-12 on the number of salivary mutans streptococci and lacto-bacilli. *Acta Odontol Scand.* 2008 Jun;66(3):154-8.

Campieri C, Campieri M, Bertuzzi V, Swennen E, Matteuzzi D, Stefoni S, Pirovano F, Centi C, Ulisse S, Famularo G, De Simone C. Reduction of oxaluria after an oral course of lactic acid bacteria at high concentration. *Kidney Int.* 2001 Sep;60(3):1097-105.

Canani RB, Cirillo P, Terrin G, Cesarano L, Spagnuolo MI, De Vincenzo A, Albano F, Passariello A, De Marco G, Manguso F, Guarino A. Probiotics for treatment of acute diarrhoea in children: randomised clinical trial of five different preparations. *BMJ.* 2007 Aug 18;335(7615):340.

Canducci F, Armuzzi A, Cremonini F, Cammarota G, Bartolozzi F, Pola P, Gasbarrini G, Gasbarrini A. A lyophilized and inactivated culture of *Lactobacillus acidophilus* increases *Helicobacter pylori* eradication rates. *Aliment Pharmacol Ther.* 2000 Dec;14(12):1625-9.

Canducci F, Cremonini F, Armuzzi A, Di Caro S, Gabrielli M, Santarelli L, Nista E, Lupascu A, De Martini D, Gasbarrini A. Probiotics and *Helicobacter pylori* eradication. *Dig Liver Dis.* 2002 Sep;34 Suppl 2:S81-3.

Carpita N. C., Kanabus J., Housley T. L. Linkage structure of fructans and fructan oligomers from Triticum aestivum and Festuca arundinacea leaves. *J. Plant Physiol.* 1989;134:162-168

Cats A, Kuipers EJ, Bosschaert MA, Pot RG, Vandenbroucke-Grauls CM, Kusters JG. Effect of frequent consumption of a *Lactobacillus casei*-containing milk drink in *Helicobacter pylori*-colonized subjects. *Aliment Pharmacol Ther.* 2003 Feb;17(3):429-35.

Chaitow L, Trenev N. *Probiotics: The revolutionary, friendly bacteria way to vital health and well-being.* New York: Thorsons, 1990.

Chao A, Thun MJ, Connell CJ, McCullough ML, Jacobs EJ, Flanders WD, Rodriguez C, Sinha R, Calle EE. Meat consumption and risk of colorectal cancer. *JAMA.* 2005 Jan 12;293(2):172-82.

Chapat L, Chemin K, Dubois B, Bourdet-Sicard R, Kaiserlian D. *Lactobacillus casei* reduces CD8+ T cell-mediated skin inflammation. *Eur J Immunol.* 2004 Sep;34(9):2520-8.

Chiang BL, Sheih YH, Wang LH, Liao CK, Gill HS. Enhancing immunity by dietary consumption of a probiotic lactic acid bacterium (*Bifidobacterium lactis* HN019): optimization and definition of cellular immune responses. *Eur J Clin Nutr.* 2000 Nov;54(11):849-55.

Chilton F, Tucker L. *Win the War Within.* New York: Rodale, 2006.

Chouraqui JP, Grathwohl D, Labaune JM, Hascoet JM, de Montgolfier I, Leclaire M, Giarre M, Steenhout P. Assessment of the safety, tolerance, and protective effect against diarrhea of infant formulas containing mixtures of probiotics or probiotics and prebiotics in a randomized controlled trial. *Am J Clin Nutr.* 2008 May;87(5):1365-73.

Chouraqui JP, Van Egroo LD, Fichot MC. Acidified milk formula supplemented with *Bifidobacterium lactis*: impact on infant diarrhea in residential care settings. *J Pediatr Gastroenterol Nutr.* 2004 Mar;38(3):288-92.

Chwirot WB, Popp F. White-light-induced luminescence and mitotic activity of yeast cells. *Folia Histochemica et Cytobiologica.* 1991;29(4):155.

Cianci A, Giordano R, Delia A, Grasso E, Amodeo A, De Leo V, Caccamo F. Efficacy of *Lactobacillus rhamnosus* GR-1 and of *Lactobacillus reuteri* RC-14 in the treatment and prevention of vaginoses and bacterial vaginitis relapses. *Minerva Ginecol.* 2008 Oct;60(5):369-76.

Clerici M, Balotta C, Meroni L, Ferrario E, Riva C, Trabattoni D, Ridolfo A, Villa M, Shearer GM, Moroni M, Galli M. Type 1 cytokine production and low prevalence of viral isolation correlate with long-term nonprogression in HIV infection. *AIDS Res Hum Retroviruses.* 1996 Jul 20;12(11):1053-61.

Cobo Sanz JM, Mateos JA, Muñoz Conejo A. Effect of *Lactobacillus casei* on the incidence of infectious conditions in children. *Nutr Hosp.* 2006 Jul-Aug;21(4):547-51.

Cohen S, Popp F. Biophoton emission of the human body. *J Photochem & Photobio.* 1997;B 40:187-189.

Colecchia A, Vestito A, La Rocca A, Pasqui F, Nikiforaki A, Festi D; Symbiotic Study Group. Effect of a symbiotic preparation on the clinical manifestations of irritable bowel syndrome, constipation-variant. Results of an open, uncontrolled multicenter study. *Minerva Gastroenterol Dietol.* 2006 Dec;52(4):349-58.

Colodner R, Edelstein H, Chazan B, Raz R. Vaginal colonization by orally administered *Lactobacillus rhamnosus* GG. *Isr Med Assoc J.* 2003 Nov;5(11):767-9.

Consumer Reports. Probiotics: Are enough in your diet? *Cons Rpts Mag.* 2005:34-35.

Conway PL, Gorbach SL, Goldin BR. Survival of lactic acid bacteria in the human stomach and adhesion to intestinal cells. *J Dairy Sci.* 1987 Jan;70(1):1-12.

Corrêa NB, Péret Filho LA, Penna FJ, Lima FM, Nicoli JR. A randomized formula controlled trial of *Bifidobacterium lactis* and *Streptococcus thermophilus* for prevention of antibiotic-associated diarrhea in infants. *J Clin Gastroenterol.* 2005 May-Jun;39(5):385-9.

Cosseau C, Devine DA, Dullaghan E, Gardy JL, Chikatamarla A, Gellatly S, Yu LL, Pistolic J, Falsafi R, Tagg J, Hancock RE. The commensal Streptococcus salivarius K12 downregulates the innate immune responses of human epithelial cells and promotes host-microbe homeostasis. *Infect Immun.* 2008 Sep;76(9):4163-75.

Dalaly BK, Eitenmiller RR, Friend BA, Shahani KM. Human milk ribonuclease. *Biochim Biophys Acta.* 1980 Oct;615(2):381-91.

Dalaly BK, Eitenmiller RR, Vakil JR, Shahani KM. Simultaneous isolation of human milk ribonuclease and lysozyme. *Anal Biochem.* 1970 Sep;37(1):208-11.

De Preter V, Raemen H, Cloetens L, Houben E, Rutgeerts P, Verbeke K. Effect of dietary intervention with different pre- and probiotics on intestinal bacterial enzyme activities. *Eur J Clin Nutr.* 2008 Feb;62(2):225-31.

De Simone C, Ciardi A, Grassi A, Lambert Gardini S, Tzantzoglou S, Trinchieri V, Moretti S, Jirillo E. Effect of *Bifidobacterium bifidum* and *Lactobacillus acidophilus* on gut mucosa and peripheral blood B lymphocytes. *Immunopharmacol Immunotoxicol.* 1992;14(1-2):331-40.

de Vrese M, Rautenberg P, Laue C, Koopmans M, Herremans T, Schrezenmeir J. Probiotic bacteria stimulate virus-specific neutralizing antibodies following a booster polio vaccination. *Eur J Nutr.* 2005 Oct;44(7):406-13.

de Vrese M, Winkler P, Rautenberg P, Harder T, Noah C, Laue C, Ott S, Hampe J, Schreiber S, Heller K, Schrezenmeir J. Effect of *Lactobacillus gasseri* PA 16/8, *Bifidobacterium longum* SP 07/3, B. *bifidum* MF 20/5 on common cold episodes: a double blind, randomized, controlled trial. *Clin Nutr.* 2005 Aug;24(4):481-91.

Dean C. *Death by Modern Medicine.* Belleville, ON: Matrix Verite-Media, 2005.

Delia A, Morgante G, Rago G, Musacchio MC, Petraglia F, De Leo V. Effectiveness of oral administration of *Lactobacillus paracasei* subsp. paracasei F19 in association with vaginal suppositories of *Lactobacillus acidofilus* in the treatment of vaginosis and in the prevention of recurrent vaginitis. *Minerva Ginecol.* 2006 Jun;58(3):227-31.

DeMan, JC, Rogosa M, Sharpe ME. A medium for the cultivation of lactobacilli. *J Bacteriol.* 1960:23;130.

Denys GA, Koch KM, Dowzicky MJ. Distribution of resistant gram-positive organisms across the census regions of the United States and in vitro activity of tigecycline, a new glycylcycline antimicrobial. *Am J Infect Control.* 2007 Oct;35(8):521-6.

Depeint F, Tzortzis G, Vulevic J, I'anson K, Gibson GR. Prebiotic evaluation of a novel galactooligosaccharide mixture produced by the enzymatic activity of *Bifidobacterium bifidum* NCIMB 41171, in healthy humans: a randomized, double-blind, crossover, placebo-controlled intervention study. *Am J Clin Nutr.* 2008 Mar;87(3):785-91.

Desbonnet L, Garrett L, Clarke G, Bienenstock J, Dinan TG. The probiotic Bifidobacteria infantis: An assessment of potential antidepressant properties in the rat. *J Psychiatr Res.* 2008 Dec;43(2):164-74.

DeWitt RC, Kudsk KA. The gut's role in metabolism, mucosal barrier function, and gut immunology. *Infect Dis Clin North Am.* 1999 Jun;13(2):465-81.

Di Marzio L, Centi C, Cinque B, Masci S, Giuliani M, Arcieri A, Zicari L, De Simone C, Cifone MG. Effect of the lactic acid bacterium *Streptococcus thermophilus* on stratum corneum ceramide levels and signs and symptoms of atopic dermatitis patients. *Exp Dermatol.* 2003 Oct;12(5):615-20.

Dierksen KP, Moore CJ, Inglis M, Wescombe PA, Tagg JR. The effect of ingestion of milk supplemented with salivaricin A-producing Streptococcus salivarius on the bacteriocin-like inhibitory activity of streptococcal populations on the tongue. *FEMS Microbiol Ecol.* 2007 Mar;59(3):584-91.

Dimitonova SP, Danova ST, Serkedjieva JP, Bakalov BV. Antimicrobial activity and protective properties of vaginal lactobacilli from healthy Bulgarian women. *Anaerobe.* 2007 Oct-Dec;13(5-6):178-84.

Dinleyici EC, Eren M, Yargic ZA, Dogan N, Vandenplas Y. Clinical efficacy of *Saccharomyces boulardii* and metronidazole compared to metronidazole alone in children with acute bloody diarrhea caused by amebiasis: a prospective, randomized, open label study. *Am J Trop Med Hyg.* 2009 Jun;80(6):953-5.

Diop L, Guillou S, Durand H. Probiotic food supplement reduces stress-induced gastrointestinal symptoms in volunteers: a double-blind, placebo-controlled, randomized trial. *Nutr Res.* 2008 Jan;28(1):1-5.

Dotolo Institute. *The Study of Colon Hydrotherapy.* Pinellas Park, FL: Dotolo, 2003.

Drago L, De Vecchi E, Nicola L, Zucchetti E, Gismondo MR, Vicariotto F. Activity of a *Lactobacillus acidophilus*-based douche for the treatment of bacterial vaginosis. *J Altern Complement Med.* 2007 May;13(4):435-8.

Drouault-Holowacz S, Bieuvelet S, Burckel A, Cazaubiel M, Dray X, Marteau P. A double blind randomized controlled trial of a probiotic combination in 100 patients with irritable bowel syndrome. *Gastroenterol Clin Biol.* 2008 Feb;32(2):147-52.

Elmer GW, McFarland LV, Surawicz CM, Danko L, Greenberg RN. Behaviour of *Saccharomyces boulardii* in recurrent *Clostridium difficile* disease patients. *Aliment Pharmacol Ther.* 1999 Dec;13(12):1663-8.

Fabian E, Elmadfa I. Influence of daily consumption of probiotic and conventional yoghurt on the plasma lipid profile in young healthy women. *Ann Nutr Metab.* 2006;50(4):387-93.

Fabian E, Majchrzak D, Dieminger B, Meyer E, Elmadfa I. Influence of probiotic and conventional yoghurt on the status of vitamins B1, B2 and B6 in young healthy women. *Ann Nutr Metab.* 2008;52(1):29-36.

Fang H, Elina T, Heikki A, Seppo S. Modulation of humoral immune response through probiotic intake. *FEMS Immunol Med Microbiol.* 2000 Sep;29(1):47-52.

Fanigliulo L, Comparato G, Aragona G, Cavallaro L, Iori V, Maino M, Cavestro GM, Soliani P, Sianesi M, Franzè A, Di Mario F. Role of gut microflora and probiotic effects in the irritable bowel syndrome. *Acta Biomed.* 2006 Aug;77(2):85-9.

Farber JE, Ross J, Stephens G. Antibiotic anaphylaxis. *Calif Med.* 1954 Jul;81(1):9-11.

Farber JE, Ross J. Antibiotic anaphylaxis; a note on the treatment and prevention of severe reactions to penicillin, streptomycin and dihydrostreptomycin. *Med Times.* 1952 Jan;80(1):28-30.

Fasano A, Shea-Donohue T. Mechanisms of disease: the role of intestinal barrier function in the pathogenesis of gastrointestinal autoimmune diseases. *Nat Clin Pract Gastroenterol Hepatol.* 2005 Sep;2(9):416-22.

Felley CP, Corthésy-Theulaz I, Rivero JL, Sipponen P, Kaufmann M, Bauerfeind P, Wiesel PH, Brassart D, Pfeifer A, Blum AL, Michetti P. Favourable effect of an acidified milk (LC-1) on *Helicobacter pylori* gastritis in man. *Eur J Gastroenterol Hepatol.* 2001 Jan;13(1):25-9.

Ferencík M, Ebringer L, Mikes Z, Jahnová E, Ciznár I. Successful modification of human intestinal microflora with oral administration of lactic acid bacteria. *Bratisl Lek Listy.* 1999 May;100(5):238-45.

Ferrier L, Berard F, Debrauwer L, Chabo C, Langella P, Bueno L, Fioramonti J. Impairment of the intestinal barrier by ethanol involves enteric microflora and mast cell activation in rodents. *Am J Pathol.* 2006 Apr;168(4):1148-54.

Firmesse O, Alvaro E, Mogenet A, Bresson JL, Lemée R, Le Ruyet P, Bonhomme C, Lambert D, Andrieux C, Doré J, Corthier G, Furet JP, Rigottier-Gois L. Fate and effects of Camembert cheese microorganisms in the human colonic microbiota of healthy volunteers after regular Camembert consumption. *Int J Food Microbiol.* 2008 Jul 15;125(2):176-81.

Forestier C, Guelon D, Cluytens V, Gillart T, Sirot J, De Champs C. Oral probiotic and prevention of *Pseudomonas aeruginosa* infections: a randomized, double-blind, placebo-controlled pilot study in intensive care unit patients. *Crit Care.* 2008;12(3):R69.

Francavilla R, Lionetti E, Castellaneta SP, Magistà AM, Maurogiovanni G, Bucci N, De Canio A, Indrio F, Cavallo L, Ierardi E, Miniello VL. Inhibition of *Helicobacter pylori* infection in humans by *Lactobacillus reuteri* ATCC 55730 and effect on eradication therapy: a pilot study. *Helicobacter.* 2008 Apr;13(2):127-34.

Friend BA, Shahani KM, Long CA, Vaughn LA. The effect of processing and storage on key enzymes, B vitamins, and lipids of mature human milk. Evaluation of fresh samples and effects of freezing and frozen storage. *Pediatr Res.* 1983 Jan;17(1):61-4.

Friend BA, Shahani KM. Characterization and evaluation of Aspergillus oryzae lactase coupled to a regenerable support. *Biotechnol Bioeng.* 1982 Feb;24(2):329-45.

Fujii T, Ohtsuka Y, Lee T, Kudo T, Shoji H, Sato H, Nagata S, Shimizu T, Yamashiro Y. *Bifidobacterium breve* enhances transforming growth factor beta1 signaling by regulating Smad7 expression in preterm infants. *J Pediatr Gastroenterol Nutr.* 2006 Jul;43(1):83-8.

Fujimori S, Gudis K, Mitsui K, Seo T, Yonezawa M, Tanaka S, Tatsuguchi A, Sakamoto C. A randomized controlled trial on the efficacy of synbiotic versus probiotic or prebiotic treatment to improve the quality of life in patients with ulcerative colitis. *Nutrition.* 2009 May;25(5):520-5.

Furrie E, Macfarlane S, Kennedy A, Cummings JH, Walsh SV, O'neil DA, Macfarlane GT. Synbiotic therapy (*Bifidobacterium longum*/Synergy 1) initiates resolution of inflammation in patients with active ulcerative colitis: a randomised controlled pilot trial. *Gut.* 2005 Feb;54(2):242-9.

Gaón D, Doweck Y, Gómez Zavaglia A, Ruiz Holgado A, Oliver G. Lactose digestion by milk fermented with *Lactobacillus acidophilus* and *Lactobacillus casei* of human origin. *Medicina (B Aires).* 1995;55(3):237-42.

Gaón D, García H, Winter L, Rodríguez N, Quintás R, González SN, Oliver G. Effect of *Lactobacillus* strains and *Saccharomyces boulardii* on persistent diarrhea in children. *Medicina (B Aires).* 2003;63(4):293-8.

ORAL PROBIOTICS

Gaón D, Garmendia C, Murrielo NO, de Cucco Games A, Cerchio A, Quintas R, González SN, Oliver G. Effect of *Lactobacillus* strains (*L. casei* and *L. Acidophilus* Strains cerela) on bacterial overgrowth-related chronic diarrhea. *Medicina.* 2002;62(2):159-63.

Garcia Vilela E, De Lourdes De Abreu Ferrari M, Oswaldo Da Gama Torres H, Guerra Pinto A, Carolina Carneiro Aguirre A, Paiva Martins F, Marcos Andrade Goulart E, Sales Da Cunha A. Influence of *Saccharomyces boulardii* on the intestinal permeability of patients with Crohn's disease in remission. *Scand J Gastroenterol.* 2008;43(7):842-8.

Gawrońska A, Dziechciarz P, Horvath A, Szajewska H. A randomized double-blind placebo-controlled trial of *Lactobacillus* GG for abdominal pain disorders in children. *Aliment Pharmacol Ther.* 2007 Jan 15;25(2):177-84.

Gill HS, Rutherfurd KJ, Cross ML, Gopal PK. Enhancement of immunity in the elderly by dietary supplementation with the probiotic *Bifidobacterium lactis* HN019. *Am J Clin Nutr.* 2001 Dec;74(6):833-9.

Gill HS, Rutherfurd KJ, Cross ML. Dietary probiotic supplementation enhances natural killer cell activity in the elderly: an investigation of age-related immunological changes. *J Clin Immunol.* 2001 Jul;21(4):264-71.

Gionchetti P, Rizzello F, Venturi A, Brigidi P, Matteuzzi D, Bazzocchi G, Poggioli G, Miglioli M, Campieri M. Oral bacteriotherapy as maintenance treatment in patients with chronic pouchitis: a double-blind, placebo-controlled trial. *Gastroenterology.* 2000 Aug;119(2):305-9.

Gittleman AL. *Guess What Came to Dinner.* New York: Avery, 2001.

Glück U, Gebbers J. Ingested probiotics reduce nasal colonization with pathogenic bacteria (*Staphylococcus aureus, Streptococcus pneumoniae,* and b-hemolytic streptococci. *Am J. Clin. Nutr.* 2003;77:517-520.

Goldin BR, Adlercreutz H, Gorbach SL, Warram JH, Dwyer JT, Swenson L, Woods MN. Estrogen excretion patterns and plasma levels in vegetarian and omnivorous women. *N Engl J Med.* 1982 Dec 16;307(25):1542-7.

Goldin BR, Swenson L, Dwyer J, Sexton M, Gorbach SL. Effect of diet and *Lactobacillus acidophilus* supplements on human fecal bacterial enzymes. *J Natl Cancer Inst.* 1980 Feb;64(2):255-61.

Goossens D, Jonkers D, Russel M, Stobberingh E, Van Den Bogaard A, StockbrUgger R. The effect of *Lactobacillus plantarum* 299v on the bacterial composition and metabolic activity in faeces of healthy volunteers: a placebo-controlled study on the onset and duration of effects. *Aliment Pharmacol Ther.* 2003 Sep 1;18(5):495-505.

Goossens DA, Jonkers DM, Russel MG, Stobberingh EE, Stockbrügger RW. The effect of a probiotic drink with *Lactobacillus plantarum* 299v on the bacterial composition in faeces and mucosal biopsies of rectum and ascending colon. *Aliment Pharmacol Ther.* 2006 Jan 15;23(2):255-63.

Gotteland M, Poliak L, Cruchet S, Brunser O. Effect of regular ingestion of *Saccharomyces boulardii* plus inulin or *Lactobacillus acidophilus* LB in children colonized by *Helicobacter pylori. Acta Paediatr.* 2005 Dec;94(12):1747-51.

Grasso F, Grillo C, Musumeci F, Triglia A, Rodolico G, Cammisuli F, Rinzivillo C, Fragati G, Santuccio A, Rodolico M. Photon emission from normal and tumour human tissues. *Experientia.* 1992;48:10-13.

Grönlund MM, Gueimonde M, Laitinen K, Kociubinski G, Grönroos T, Salminen S, Isolauri E. Maternal breast-milk and intestinal bifidobacteria guide the compositional development of the *Bifidobacterium* microbiota in infants at risk of allergic disease. *Clin Exp Allergy.* 2007 Dec;37(12):1764-72.

Groppo FC, Ramacciato JC, Simões RP, Flório FM, Sartoratto A. Antimicrobial activity of garlic, tea tree oil, and chlorhexidine against oral microorganisms. *Int Dent J.* 2002 Dec;52(6):433-7.

Guarino A, Canani RB, Spagnuolo MI, Albano F, Di Benedetto L. Oral bacterial therapy reduces the duration of symptoms and of viral excretion in children with mild diarrhea. *J Pediatr Gastroenterol Nutr.* 1997 Nov;25(5):516-9.

Guerin-Danan C, Chabanet C, Pedone C, Popot F, Vaissade P, Bouley C, Szylit O, Andrieux C. Milk fermented with yogurt cultures and *Lactobacillus casei* compared with yogurt and gelled milk: influence on intestinal microflora in healthy infants. *Am J Clin Nutr.* 1998 Jan;67(1):111-7.

Guslandi M, Giollo P, Testoni PA. A pilot trial of *Saccharomyces boulardii* in ulcerative colitis. *Eur J Gastroenterol Hepatol.* 2003 Jun;15(6):697-8.

Guslandi M, Mezzi G, Sorghi M, Testoni PA. *Saccharomyces boulardii* in maintenance treatment of Crohn's disease. *Dig Dis Sci.* 2000 Jul;45(7):1462-4.

Haarman M, Knol J. Quantitative real-time PCR assays to identify and quantify fecal *Bifidobacterium* species in infants receiving a prebiotic infant formula. Appl Environ Microbiol. 2005 May;71(5):2318-24.

Hallén A, Jarstrand C, Påhlson C. Treatment of bacterial vaginosis with lactobacilli. Sex Transm Dis. 1992 May-Jun;19(3):146-8.

Harris LA, Chang L. Irritable bowel syndrome: new and emerging therapies. *Curr Opin Gastroenterol.* 2006 Mar;22(2):128-35.

Harvey HP, Solomon HJ. Acute anaphylactic shock due to para-aminosalicylic acid. *Am Rev Tuberc.* 1958 Mar;77(3):492-5.

REFERENCES AND BIBLIOGRAPHY

Hata Y, Yamamoto M, Ohni M, Nakajima K, Nakamura Y, Takano T. A placebo-controlled study of the effect of sour milk on blood pressure in hypertensive subjects. *Am J Clin Nutr.* 1996 Nov;64(5):767-71.

Hatakka K, Holma R, El-Nezami H, Suomalainen T, Kuisma M, Saxelin M, Poussa T, Mykkänen H, Korpela R. The influence of *Lactobacillus rhamnosus* LC705 together with Propionibacterium freudenreichii ssp. shermanii JS on potentially carcinogenic bacterial activity in human colon. *Int J Food Microbiol.* 2008 Dec 10;128(2):406-10.

Hattori K, Yamamoto A, Sasai M, Taniuchi S, Kojima T, Kobayashi Y, Iwamoto H, Namba K, Yaeshima T. Effects of administration of bifidobacteria on fecal microflora and clinical symptoms in infants with atopic dermatitis. *Arerugi.* 2003 Jan;52(1):20-30.

He M, Antoine JM, Yang Y, Yang J, Men J, Han H. Influence of live flora on lactose digestion in male adult lactose-malabsorbers after dairy products intake. *Wei Sheng Yan Jiu.* 2004 Sep;33(5):603-5.

He T, Priebe MG, Zhong Y, Huang C, Harmsen HJ, Raangs GC, Antoine JM, Welling GW, Vonk RJ. Effects of yogurt and bifidobacteria supplementation on the colonic microbiota in lactose-intolerant subjects. *J Appl Microbiol.* 2008 Feb;104(2):595-604.

Hickson M, D'Souza AL, Muthu N, Rogers TR, Want S, Rajkumar C, Bulpitt CJ. Use of probiotic *Lactobacillus* preparation to prevent diarrhoea associated with antibiotics: randomised double blind placebo controlled trial. *BMJ.* 2007 Jul 14;335(7610):80.

Hillman JD, McDonell E, Cramm T, Hillman CH, Zahradnik RT. A spontaneous lactate dehydrogenase deficient mutant of Streptococcus rattus for use as a probiotic in the prevention of dental caries. *J Appl Microbiol.* 2009 Nov;107(5):1551-8.

Hillman JD, McDonell E, Hillman CH, Zahradnik RT, Soni MG. Safety assessment of ProBiora3, a probiotic mouthwash: subchronic toxicity study in rats. *Int J Toxicol.* 2009 Sep-Oct;28(5):357-67.

Hilton E, Isenberg HD, Alperstein P, France K, Borenstein MT. Ingestion of yogurt containing *Lactobacillus acidophilus* as prophylaxis for *Candida* vaginitis. *Ann Intern Med.* 1992 Mar 1;116(5):353-7.

Hirose Y, Murosaki S, Yamamoto Y, Yoshikai Y, Tsuru T. Daily intake of heat-killed *Lactobacillus plantarum* L-137 augments acquired immunity in healthy adults. *J Nutr.* 2006 Dec;136(12):3069-73.

Hlivak P, Jahnova E, Odraska J, Ferencik M, Ebringer L, Mikes Z. Long-term (56-week) oral administration of probiotic *Enterococcus faecium* M-74 decreases the expression of sICAM-1 and monocyte CD54, and increases that of lymphocyte CD49d in humans. *Bratisl Lek Listy.* 2005;106(4-5):175-81.

Hlivak P, Odraska J, Ferencik M, Ebringer L, Jahnova E, Mikes Z. One-year application of probiotic strain *Enterococcus faecium* M-74 decreases serum cholesterol levels. *Bratisl Lek Listy.* 2005;106(2):67-72.

Hobbs C. *Kombucha Manchurian Tea Mushroom: The Essential Guide.* Santa Cruz, CA: Botanica Press, 1995.

Hobbs C. *Stress & Natural Healing.* Loveland, CO: Interweave Press, 1997.

Horz HP, Meinelt A, Houben B, Conrads G. Distribution and persistence of probiotic Streptococcus salivarius K12 in the human oral cavity as determined by real-time quantitative polymerase chain reaction. *Oral Microbiol Immunol.* 2007 Apr;22(2):126-30.

Hota B, Ellenbogen C, Hayden MK, Aroutcheva A, Rice TW, Weinstein RA. Community-associated methicillin-resistant *Staphylococcus aureus* skin and soft tissue infections at a public hospital: do public housing and incarceration amplify transmission? *Arch Intern Med.* 2007 May 28;167(10):1026-33.

Hoyme UB, Saling E. Efficient prematurity prevention is possible by pH-self measurement and immediate therapy of threatening ascending infection. *Eur J Obstet Gynecol Reprod Biol.* 2004 Aug 10;115(2):148-53.

Hoyos AB. Reduced incidence of necrotizing enterocolitis associated with enteral administration of *Lactobacillus acidophilus* and *Bifidobacterium infantis* to neonates in an intensive care unit. *Int J Infect Dis.* 1999 Summer;3(4):197-202.

Humphrey LL, Fu R, Buckley DI, Freeman M, Helfand M. Periodontal disease and coronary heart disease incidence: a systematic review and meta-analysis. *J Gen Intern Med.* 2008 Dec;23(12):2079-86.

Hun L. Bacillus coagulans significantly improved abdominal pain and bloating in patients with IBS. *Postgrad Med.* 2009 Mar;121(2):119-24.

Hyink O, Wescombe PA, Upton M, Ragland N, Burton JP, Tagg JR. Salivaricin A2 and the novel lantibiotic salivaricin B are encoded at adjacent loci on a 190-kilobase transmissible megaplasmid in the oral probiotic strain Streptococcus salivarius K12. *Appl Environ Microbiol.* 2007 Feb;73(4):1107-13.

Iakovenko VD, Filatov VF, Dikiĭ IL. The cause-effect interdependence in the pathogenesis of chronic tonsillitis as an infectious allergic process. *Vestn Otorinolaringol.* 1990 Mar-Apr;(2):52-6.

Imase K, Tanaka A, Tokunaga K, Sugano H, Ishida H, Takahashi S. *Lactobacillus reuteri* tablets suppress *Helicobacter pylori* infection—a double-blind randomised placebo-controlled cross-over clinical study. *Kansenshogaku Zasshi.* 2007 Jul;81(4):387-93.

Indrio F, Ladisa G, Mautone A, Montagna O. Effect of a fermented formula on thymus size and stool pH in healthy term infants. *Pediatr Res.* 2007 Jul;62(1):98-100.

Indrio F, Riezzo G, Raimondi F, Bisceglia M, Cavallo L, Francavilla R. The effects of probiotics on feeding tolerance, bowel habits, and gastrointestinal motility in preterm newborns. *J Pediatr.* 2008 Jun;152(6):801-6.

Iovieno A, Lambiase A, Sacchetti M, Stampachiacchiere B, Micera A, Bonini S. Preliminary evidence of the efficacy of probiotic eye-drop treatment in patients with vernal keratoconjunctivitis. *Graefes Arch Clin Exp Ophthalmol.* 2008 Mar;246(3):435-41.

Ishida Y, Nakamura F, Kanzato H, Sawada D, Hirata H, Nishimura A, Kajimoto O, Fujiwara S. Clinical effects of *Lactobacillus acidophilus* strain L-92 on perennial allergic rhinitis: a double-blind, placebo-controlled study. *J Dairy Sci.* 2005 Feb;88(2):527-33.

Ishida Y, Nakamura F, Kanzato H, Sawada D, Yamamoto N, Kagata H, Oh-Ida M, Takeuchi H, Fujiwara S. Effect of milk fermented with *Lactobacillus acidophilus* strain L-92 on symptoms of Japanese cedar pollen allergy: a randomized placebo-controlled trial. *Biosci Biotechnol Biochem.* 2005 Sep;69(9):1652-60.

Ishikawa H, Akedo I, Otani T, Suzuki T, Nakamura T, Takeyama I, Ishiguro S, Miyaoka E, Sobue T, Kakizoe T. Randomized trial of dietary fiber and *Lactobacillus casei* administration for prevention of colorectal tumors. *Int J Cancer.* 2005 Sep 20;116(5):762-7.

Isolauri E, Joensuu J, Suomalainen H, Luomala M, Vesikari T. Improved immunogenicity of oral D x RRV reassortant rotavirus vaccine by *Lactobacillus casei* GG. *Vaccine.* 1995 Feb;13(3):310-2.

Isolauri E, Juntunen M, Rautanen T, Sillanaukee P, Koivula T. A human *Lactobacillus* strain (*Lactobacillus casei* sp strain GG) promotes recovery from acute diarrhea in children. *Pediatrics.* 1991 Jul;88(1):90-7.

Isolauri E, Kaila M, Mykkänen H, Ling WH, Salminen S. Oral bacteriotherapy for viral gastroenteritis. *Dig Dis Sci.* 1994 Dec;39(12):2595-600.

Ivory K, Chambers SJ, Pin C, Prieto E, Arqués JL, Nicoletti C. Oral delivery of *Lactobacillus casei* Shirota modifies allergen-induced immune responses in allergic rhinitis. *Clin Exp Allergy.* 2008 Aug;38(8):1282-9.

Jacobsen CN, Rosenfeldt Nielsen V, Hayford AE, Moller PL, Michaelsen KF, Paerregaard A, Sandström B, Tvede M, Jakobsen M. Screening of probiotic activities of forty-seven strains of *Lactobacillus* spp. by in vitro techniques and evaluation of the colonization ability of five selected strains in humans. *Appl Environ Microbiol.* 1999 Nov;65(11):4949-56.

Jain PK, McNaught CE, Anderson AD, MacFie J, Mitchell CJ. Influence of synbiotic containing *Lactobacillus acidophilus* La5, *Bifidobacterium lactis* Bb 12, *Streptococcus thermophilus*, *Lactobacillus bulgaricus* and oligofructose on gut barrier function and sepsis in critically ill patients: a randomised controlled trial. *Clin Nutr.* 2004 Aug;23(4):467-75.

Janelle KC, Barr SI. Nutrient intakes and eating behavior scores of vegetarian and nonvegetarian women. *J Am Diet Assoc.* 1995 Feb;95(2):180-6, 189, quiz 187-8.

Jauhiainen T, Vapaatalo H, Poussa T, Kyrönpalo S, Rasmussen M, Korpela R. *Lactobacillus helveticus* fermented milk lowers blood pressure in hypertensive subjects in 24-h ambulatory blood pressure measurement. *Am J Hypertens.* 2005 Dec;18(12 Pt 1):1600-5.

Jensen B. *Foods that Heal.* Garden City Park, NY: Avery Publ, 1988, 1993.

Jiang T, Mustapha A, Savaiano DA. Improvement of lactose digestion in humans by ingestion of unfermented milk containing *Bifidobacterium longum*. *J Dairy Sci.* 1996 May;79(5):750-7.

Jiménez E, Fernández L, Maldonado A, Martín R, Olivares M, Xaus J, Rodríguez JM. Oral administration of *Lactobacillus* strains isolated from breast milk as an alternative for the treatment of infectious mastitis during lactation. *Appl Environ Microbiol.* 2008 Aug;74(15):4650-5.

Johansson G, Holmén A, Persson L, Högstedt B, Wassén C, Ottova L, Gustafsson JA. Dietary influence on some proposed risk factors for colon cancer: fecal and urinary mutagenic activity and the activity of some intestinal bacterial enzymes. *Cancer Detect Prev.* 1997;21(3):258-66.

Johansson GK, Ottova L, Gustafsson JA. Shift from a mixed diet to a lactovegetarian diet: influence on some cancer-associated intestinal bacterial enzyme activities. *Nutr Cancer.* 1990;14(3-4):239-46. PubMed PMID: 2128119.

Johansson ML, Nobaek S, Berggren A, Nyman M, Björck I, Ahrné S, Jeppsson B, Molin G. Survival of *Lactobacillus plantarum* DSM 9843 (299v), and effect on the short-chain fatty acid content of faeces after ingestion of a rose-hip drink with fermented oats. *Int J Food Microbiol.* 1998 Jun 30;42(1-2):29-38.

Jones SE, Versalovic J. Probiotic *Lactobacillus reuteri* biofilms produce antimicrobial and anti-inflammatory factors. *BMC Microbiol.* 2009 Feb 11;9:35.

Kaila M, Isolauri E, Saxelin M, Arvilommi H, Vesikari T. Viable versus inactivated *Lactobacillus* strain GG in acute rotavirus diarrhoea. *Arch Dis Child.* 1995 Jan;72(1):51-3.

Kajander K, Hatakka K, Poussa T, Färkkilä M, Korpela R. A probiotic mixture alleviates symptoms in irritable bowel syndrome patients: a controlled 6-month intervention. *Aliment Pharmacol Ther.* 2005 Sep 1;22(5):387-94.

Kajander K, Korpela R. Clinical studies on alleviating the symptoms of irritable bowel syndrome. *Asia Pac J Clin Nutr.* 2006;15(4):576-80.

Kajander K, Krogius-Kurikka L, Rinttilä T, Karjalainen H, Palva A, Korpela R. Effects of multispecies probiotic supplementation on intestinal microbiota in irritable bowel syndrome. *Aliment Pharmacol Ther.* 2007 Aug 1;26(3):463-73.

REFERENCES AND BIBLIOGRAPHY

Kajander K, Myllyluoma E, Rajilić-Stojanović M, Kyrönpalo S, Rasmussen M, Järvenpää S, Zoetendal EG, de Vos WM, Vapaatalo H, Korpela R. Clinical trial: multispecies probiotic supplementation alleviates the symptoms of irritable bowel syndrome and stabilizes intestinal microbiota. *Aliment Pharmacol Ther.* 2008 Jan 1;27(1):48-57.

Kalliomäki M, Salminen S, Poussa T, Arvilommi H, Isolauri E. Probiotics and prevention of atopic disease: 4-year follow-up of a randomised placebo-controlled trial. *Lancet.* 2003 May 31;361(9372):1869-71.

Kalliomäki M, Salminen S, Poussa T, Isolauri E. Probiotics during the first 7 years of life: a cumulative risk reduction of eczema in a randomized, placebo-controlled trial. *J Allergy Clin Immunol.* 2007 Apr;119(4):1019-21.

Kanazawa H, Nagino M, Kamiya S, Komatsu S, Mayumi T, Takagi K, Asahara T, Nomoto K, Tanaka R, Nimura Y. Synbiotics reduce postoperative infectious complications: a randomized controlled trial in biliary cancer patients undergoing hepatectomy. *Langenbecks Arch Surg.* 2005 Apr;390(2):104-13.

Kankaanpää PE, Yang B, Kallio HP, Isolauri E, Salminen SJ. Influence of probiotic supplemented infant formula on composition of plasma lipids in atopic infants. *J Nutr Biochem.* 2002 Jun;13(6):364-369.

Kano H, Mogami O, Uchida M. Oral administration of milk fermented with *Lactobacillus delbrueckii* ssp. bulgaricus OLL1073R-1 to DBA/1 mice inhibits secretion of proinflammatory cytokines. *Cytotechnology.* 2002 Nov;40(1-3):67-73.

Kawase M, Hashimoto H, Hosoda M, Morita H, Hosono A. Effect of administration of fermented milk containing whey protein concentrate to rats and healthy men on serum lipids and blood pressure. *J Dairy Sci.* 2000 Feb;83(2):255-63.

Kaygusuz I, Gödekmerdan A, Karlidag T, Keleş E, Yalçin S, Aral I, Yildiz M. Early stage impacts of tonsillectomy on immune functions of children. *Int J Pediatr Otorhinolaryngol.* 2003 Dec;67(12):1311-5.

Kazansky DB. MHC restriction and allogeneic immune responses. *J Immunotoxicol.* 2008 Oct;5(4):369-84.

Kecskés G, Belágyi T, Oláh A. Early jejunal nutrition with combined pre- and probiotics in acute pancreatitis—prospective, randomized, double-blind investigations. *Magy Seb.* 2003 Feb;56(1):3-8.

Kekkonen RA, Lummela N, Karjalainen H, Latvala S, Tynkkynen S, Jarvenpaa S, Kautiainen H, Julkunen I, Vapaatalo H, Korpela R. Probiotic intervention has strain-specific anti-inflammatory effects in healthy adults. *World J Gastroenterol.* 2008 Apr 7;14(13):2029-36.

Kekkonen RA, Sysi-Aho M, Seppanen-Laakso T, Julkunen I, Vapaatalo H, Oresic M, Korpela R. Effect of probiotic *Lactobacillus rhamnosus* GG intervention on global serum lipidomic profiles in healthy adults. *World J Gastroenterol.* 2008 May 28;14(20):3188-94.

Kekkonen RA, Vasankari TJ, Vuorimaa T, Haahtela T, Julkunen I, Korpela R. The effect of probiotics on respiratory infections and gastrointestinal symptoms during training in marathon runners. *Int J Sport Nutr Exerc Metab.* 2007 Aug;17(4):352-63.

Kidambi S, Patel SB. Diabetes mellitus: considerations for dentistry. *J Am Dent Assoc.* 2008 Oct;139 Suppl:8S-18S.

Kiessling G, Schneider J, Jahreis G. Long-term consumption of fermented dairy products over 6 months increases HDL cholesterol. *Eur J Clin Nutr.* 2002 Sep;56(9):843-9.

Kilara A, Shahani KM. The use of immobilized enzymes in the food industry: a review. *CRC Crit Rev Food Sci Nutr.* 1979 Dec;12(2):161-98.

Kim LS, Waters RF, Burkholder PM. Immunological activity of larch arabinogalactan and Echinacea: a preliminary, randomized, double-blind, placebo-controlled trial. *Altern Med Rev.* 2002 Apr;7(2):138-49.

Kim MN, Kim N, Lee SH, Park YS, Hwang JH, Kim JW, Jeong SH, Lee DH, Kim JS, Jung HC, Song IS. The effects of probiotics on PPI-triple therapy for *Helicobacter pylori* eradication. *Helicobacter.* 2008 Aug;13(4):261-8.

Kim YG, Moon JT, Lee KM, Chon NR, Park H. The effects of probiotics on symptoms of irritable bowel syndrome. *Korean J Gastroenterol.* 2006 Jun;47(6):413-9.

Kinross JM, von Roon AC, Holmes E, Darzi A, Nicholson JK. The human gut microbiome: implications for future health care. *Curr Gastroenterol Rep.* 2008 Aug;10(4):396-403.

Kirjavainen PV, Arvola T, Salminen SJ, Isolauri E. Aberrant composition of gut microbiota of allergic infants: a target of bifidobacterial therapy at weaning? *Gut.* 2002 Jul;51(1):51-5.

Kirpich IA, Solovieva NV, Leikhter SN, Shidakova NA, Lebedeva OV, Sidorov PI, Bazhukova TA, Soloviev AG, Barve SS, McClain CJ, Cave M. Probiotics restore bowel flora and improve liver enzymes in human alcohol-induced liver injury: a pilot study. *Alcohol.* 2008 Dec;42(8):675-82.

Kitajima H, Sumida Y, Tanaka R, Yuki N, Takayama H, Fujimura M. Early administration of *Bifidobacterium breve* to preterm infants: randomised controlled trial. *Arch Dis Child Fetal Neonatal Ed.* 1997 Mar;76(2):F101-7.

Klarin B, Johansson ML, Molin G, Larsson A, Jeppsson B. Adhesion of the probiotic bacterium *Lactobacillus plantarum* 299v onto the gut mucosa in critically ill patients: a randomised open trial. *Crit Care.* 2005 Jun;9(3):R285-93.

Klarin B, Molin G, Jeppsson B, Larsson A. Use of the probiotic *Lactobacillus plantarum* 299 to reduce pathogenic bacteria in the oropharynx of intubated patients: a randomised controlled open pilot study. *Crit Care.* 2008;12(6):R136.

Klein A, Friedrich U, Vogelsang H, Jahreis G. *Lactobacillus acidophilus* 74-2 and *Bifidobacterium animalis* subsp *lactis* DGCC 420 modulate unspecific cellular immune response in healthy adults. *Eur J Clin Nutr.* 2008 May;62(5):584-93.

Klein E, Smith D, Laxminarayan R. Trends in Hospitalizations and Deaths in the United States Associated with Infections Caused by Staphylococcus aureus and MRSA, 1999-2004. *Emerging Infectious Diseases. University of Florida Rel.* 2007 Dec 3.

Klein U, Kanellis MJ, Drake D. Effects of four anticaries agents on lesion depth progression in an in vitro caries model. *Pediatr Dent.* 1999 May-Jun;21(3):176-80.

Klima H, Haas O, Roschger P. Photon emission from blood cells and its possible role in immune system regulation. In: Jezowska-Trzebiatowska B. (ed.): *Photon Emission from Biological Systems. Singapore: World Sci.* 1987:153-169.

Klingberg TD, Budde BB. The survival and persistence in the human gastrointestinal tract of five potential probiotic lactobacilli consumed as freeze-dried cultures or as probiotic sausage. *Int J Food Microbiol.* 2006 May 25;109(1-2):157-9.

Kloss J. *Back to Eden.* Twin Oaks, WI: Lotus Press, 1939-1999.

Kollaritsch H, Holst H, Grobara P, Wiedermann G. Prevention of traveler's diarrhea with *Saccharomyces boulardii.* Results of a placebo controlled double-blind study. *Fortschr Med.* 1993 Mar 30;111(9):152-6.

Koop H, Bachem MG. Serum iron, ferritin, and vitamin B12 during prolonged omeprazole therapy. *J Clin Gastroenterol.* 1992;14:288-92.

Korschunov VM, Smeianov VV, Efimov BA, Tarabrina NP, Ivanov AA, Baranov AE. Therapeutic use of an antibiotic-resistant *Bifidobacterium* preparation in men exposed to high-dose gamma-irradiation. *J Med Microbiol.* 1996 Jan;44(1):70-4.

Kotowska M, Albrecht P, Szajewska H. *Saccharomyces boulardii* in the prevention of antibiotic-associated diarrhoea in children: a randomized double-blind placebo-controlled trial. *Aliment Pharmacol Ther.* 2005 Mar 1;21(5):583-90.

Kotzampassi K, Giamarellos-Bourboulis EJ, Voudouris A, Kazamias P, Eleftheriadis E. Benefits of a synbiotic formula (Synbiotic 2000Forte) in critically Ill trauma patients: early results of a randomized controlled trial. *World J Surg.* 2006 Oct;30(10):1848-55.

Krasse P, Carlsson B, Dahl C, Paulsson A, Nilsson A, Sinkiewicz G. Decreased gum bleeding and reduced gingivitis by the probiotic *Lactobacillus reuteri. Swed Dent J.* 2006;30(2):55-60.

Kruger K, Kamilli I, Schattenkirchner M. Blastocystis hominis as a rare arthritogenic pathogen. *Z Rheumatol.* 1994 Mar-Apr;53(2):83-5.

Kukkonen K, Nieminen T, Poussa T, Savilahti E, Kuitunen M. Effect of probiotics on vaccine antibody responses in infancy—a randomized placebo-controlled double-blind trial. *Pediatr Allergy Immunol.* 2006 Sep;17(6):416-21.

Kukkonen K, Savilahti E, Haahtela T, Juntunen-Backman K, Korpela R, Poussa T, Tuure T, Kuitunen M. Long-term safety and impact on infection rates of postnatal probiotic and prebiotic (synbiotic) treatment: randomized, double-blind, placebo-controlled trial. *Pediatrics.* 2008 Jul;122(1):8-12.

Kukkonen K, Savilahti E, Haahtela T, Juntunen-Backman K, Korpela R, Poussa T, Tuure T, Kuitunen M. Probiotics and prebiotic galacto-oligosaccharides in the prevention of allergic diseases: a randomized, double-blind, placebo-controlled trial. *J Allergy Clin Immunol.* 2007 Jan;119(1):192-8.

Kurugöl Z, Koturoğlu G. Effects of *Saccharomyces boulardii* in children with acute diarrhoea. *Acta Paediatr.* 2005 Jan;94(1):44-7.

Kuznetsov VF, Iushchuk ND, Iurko LP, Nabokova NIu. Intestinal dysbacteriosis in yersiniosis patients and the possibility of its correction with biopreparations. *Ter Arkh.* 1994;66(11):17-8.

Laitinen K, Isolauri E. Management of food allergy: vitamins, fatty acids or probiotics? *Eur J Gastroenterol Hepatol.* 2005 Dec;17(12):1305-11.

Laitinen K, Poussa T, Isolauri E; Nutrition, Allergy, Mucosal Immunology and Intestinal Microbiota Group. Probiotics and dietary counselling contribute to glucose regulation during and after pregnancy: a randomised controlled trial. *Br J Nutr.* 2009 Jun;101(11):1679-87.

Langhendries JP, Detry J, Van Hees J, Lamboray JM, Darimont J, Mozin MJ, Secretin MC, Senterre J. Effect of a fermented infant formula containing viable bifidobacteria on the fecal flora composition and pH of healthy full-term infants. *J Pediatr Gastroenterol Nutr.* 1995 Aug;21(2):177-81.

Lara-Villoslada F, Sierra S, Boza J, Xaus J, Olivares M. Beneficial effects of consumption of a dairy product containing two probiotic strains, *Lactobacillus coryniformis* CECT5711 and *Lactobacillus gasseri* CECT5714 in healthy children. *Nutr Hosp.* 2007 Jul-Aug;22(4):496-502.

REFERENCES AND BIBLIOGRAPHY

Leal AL, Eslava-Schmalbach J, Alvarez C, Buitrago G, Méndez M; Grupo para el Control de la Resistencia Bacteriana en Bogotá. Endemic tendencies and bacterial resistance markers in third-level hospitals in Bogotá, Colombia. Rev Salud Publica (Bogota). 2006 May;8 Suppl 1:59-70.

Lee MC, Lin LH, Hung KL, Wu HY. Oral bacterial therapy promotes recovery from acute diarrhea in children. *Acta Paediatr Taiwan.* 2001 Sep-Oct;42(5):301-5.

Lee SJ, Cho SJ, Park EA. Effects of probiotics on enteric flora and feeding tolerance in preterm infants. *Neonatology.* 2007;91(3):174-9.

Lee SJ, Shim YH, Cho SJ, Lee JW. Probiotics prophylaxis in children with persistent primary vesicoureteral reflux. *Pediatr Nephrol.* 2007 Sep;22(9):1315-20.

Lee TH, Hsueh PR, Yeh WC, Wang HP, Wang TH, Lin JT. Low frequency of bacteremia after endoscopic mucosal resection. *Gastrointest Endosc.* 2000 Aug;52(2):223-5.

Lieske JC, Goldfarb DS, De Simone C, Regnier C. Use of a probiotic to decrease enteric hyperoxaluria. *Kidney Int.* 2005 Sep;68(3):1244-9.

Lin HC, Hsu CH, Chen HL, Chung MY, Hsu JF, Lien RI, Tsao LY, Chen CH, Su BH. Oral probiotics prevent necrotizing enterocolitis in very low birth weight preterm infants: a multicenter, randomized, controlled trial. *Pediatrics.* 2008 Oct;122(4):693-700.

Lin HC, Su BH, Chen AC, Lin TW, Tsai CH, Yeh TF, Oh W. Oral probiotics reduce the incidence and severity of necrotizing enterocolitis in very low birth weight infants. *Pediatrics.* 2005 Jan;115(1):1-4.

Lin JS, Chiu YH, Lin NT, Chu CH, Huang KC, Liao KW, Peng KC. Different effects of probiotic species/strains on infections in preschool children: A double-blind, randomized, controlled study. *Vaccine.* 2009 Feb 11;27(7):1073-9.

Lin SY, Ayres JW, Winkler W Jr, Sandine WE. *Lactobacillus* effects on cholesterol: in vitro and in vivo results. *J Dairy Sci.* 1989 Nov;72(11):2885-99.

Ling WH, Hänninen O. Shifting from a conventional diet to an uncooked vegan diet reversibly alters fecal hydrolytic activities in humans. *J Nutr.* 1992 Apr;122(4):924-30.

Lininger S, Gaby A, Austin S, Brown D, Wright J, Duncan A. *The Natural Pharmacy.* New York: Three Rivers, 1999.

Linsalata M, Russo F, Berloco P, Caruso ML, Matteo GD, Cifone MG, Simone CD, Ierardi E, Di Leo A. The influence of *Lactobacillus brevis* on ornithine decarboxylase activity and polyamine profiles in *Helicobacter pylori*-infected gastric mucosa. *Helicobacter.* 2004 Apr;9(2):165-72.

Lipkind M. Registration of spontaneous photon emission from virus-infected cell cultures: development of experimental system. *Indian J Exp Biol.* 2003 May;41(5):457-72.

Lipski E. *Digestive Wellness.* Los Angeles, CA: Keats, 2000.

Loguercio C, Abbiati R, Rinaldi M, Romano A, Del Vecchio Blanco C, Coltorti M. Long-term effects of *Enterococcus faecium* SF68 versus lactulose in the treatment of patients with cirrhosis and grade 1-2 hepatic encephalopathy. *J Hepatol.* 1995 Jul;23(1):39-46.

Loguercio C, Del Vecchio Blanco C, Coltorti M. Enterococcus lactic acid bacteria strain SF68 and lactulose in hepatic encephalopathy: a controlled study. *J Int Med Res.* 1987 Nov-Dec;15(6):335-43.

Lorea Baroja M, Kirjavainen PV, Hekmat S, Reid G. Anti-inflammatory effects of probiotic yogurt in inflammatory bowel disease patients. *Clin Exp Immunol.* 2007 Sep;149(3):470-9.

Lythcott GI. Anaphylaxis to viomycin. *Am Rev Tuberc.* 1957 Jan;75(1):135-8.

Madden JA, Plummer SF, Tang J, Garaiova I, Plummer NT, Herbison M, Hunter JO, Shimada T, Cheng L, Shirakawa T. Effect of probiotics on preventing disruption of the intestinal microflora following antibiotic therapy: a double-blind, placebo-controlled pilot study. *Int Immunopharmacol.* 2005 Jun;5(6):1091-7.

Mah KW, Chin VI, Wong WS, Lay C, Tannock GW, Shek LP, Aw MM, Chua KY, Wong HB, Panchalingham A, Lee BW. Effect of a milk formula containing probiotics on the fecal microbiota of asian infants at risk of atopic diseases. *Pediatr Res.* 2007 Dec;62(6):674-9.

Majamaa H, Isolauri E, Saxelin M, Vesikari T. Lactic acid bacteria in the treatment of acute rotavirus gastroenteritis. *J Pediatr Gastroenterol Nutr.* 1995 Apr;20(3):333-8.

Manley KJ, Fraenkel MB, Mayall BC, Power DA. Probiotic treatment of vancomycin-resistant enterococci: a randomised controlled trial. *Med J Aust.* 2007 May 7;186(9):454-7.

Manzoni P, Mostert M, Leonessa ML, Priolo C, Farina D, Monetti C, Latino MA, Gomirato G. Oral supplementation with *Lactobacillus casei* subspecies *rhamnosus* prevents enteric colonization by *Candida* species in preterm neonates: a randomized study. *Clin Infect Dis.* 2006 Jun 15;42(12):1735-42.

Marcos A, Wärnberg J, Nova E, Gómez S, Alvarez A, Alvarez R, Mateos JA, Cobo JM. The effect of milk fermented by yogurt cultures plus *Lactobacillus casei* DN-114001 on the immune response of subjects under academic examination stress. *Eur J Nutr.* 2004 Dec;43(6):381-9.

Marteau P, Pochart P, Bouhnik Y, Zidi S, Goderel I, Rambaud JC. Survival of *Lactobacillus acidophilus* and *Bifidobacterium* sp. in the small intestine following ingestion in fermented milk. A rational basis for the use of probiotics in man. *Gastroenterol Clin Biol.* 1992;16(1):25-8.

Martinez RC, Franceschini SA, Patta MC, Quintana SM, Candido RC, Ferreira JC, De Martinis EC, Reid G. Improved treatment of vulvovaginal candidiasis with fluconazole plus probiotic *Lactobacillus rhamnosus* GR-1 and *Lactobacillus reuteri* RC-14. *Lett Appl Microbiol.* 2009 Mar;48(3):269-74.

Martinez RC, Franceschini SA, Patta MC, Quintana SM, Gomes BC, De Martinis EC, Reid G. Improved cure of bacterial vaginosis with single dose of tinidazole (2 g), *Lactobacillus rhamnosus* GR-1, and *Lactobacillus reuteri* RC-14: a randomized, double-blind, placebo-controlled trial. *Can J Microbiol.* 2009 Feb;55(2):133-8.

Martin-Venegas R, Roig-Perez S, Ferrer R, Moreno JJ. Arachidonic acid cascade and epithelial barrier function during Caco-2 cell differentiation. *J Lipid Res.* 2006 Apr;3.

Marushko IuV. The development of a treatment method for streptococcal tonsillitis in children. *Lik Sprava.* 2000 Jan-Feb;(1):79-82.

Masuno T, Kishimoto S, Ogura T, Honma T, Niitani H, Fukuoka M, Ogawa N. A comparative trial of LC9018 plus doxorubicin and doxorubicin alone for the treatment of malignant pleural effusion secondary to lung cancer. *Cancer.* 1991 Oct 1;68(7):1495-500.

Mater DD, Bretigny L, Firmesse O, Flores MJ, Mogenet A, Bresson JL, Corthier G. *Streptococcus thermophilus* and *Lactobacillus delbrueckii* subsp. bulgaricus survive gastrointestinal transit of healthy volunteers consuming yogurt. *FEMS Microbiol Lett.* 2005 Sep 15;250(2):185-7.

Mathur BN, Shahani KM. Use of total whey constituents for human food. *J Dairy Sci.* 1979 Jan;62(1):99-105.

Matsumoto M, Benno Y. Anti-inflammatory metabolite production in the gut from the consumption of probiotic yogurt containing *Bifidobacterium animalis* subsp. *lactis* LKM512. *Biosci Biotechnol Biochem.* 2006 Jun;70(6):1287-92.

Matsumoto M, Benno Y. Consumption of *Bifidobacterium lactis* LKM512 yogurt reduces gut mutagenicity by increasing gut polyamine contents in healthy adult subjects. *Mutat Res.* 2004 Dec 21;568(2):147-53.

Matsuzaki T, Saito M, Usuku K, Nose H, Izumo S, Arimura K, Osame M. A prospective uncontrolled trial of fermented milk drink containing viable *Lactobacillus casei* strain Shirota in the treatment of HTLV-1 associated myelopathy/tropical spastic paraparesis. *J Neurol Sci.* 2005 Oct 15;237(1-2):75-81.

McDougall J, McDougall M. *The McDougal Plan.* Clinton, NJ: New Win, 1983.

McGuire BW, Sia LL, Haynes JD, Kisicki JC, Gutierrez ML, Stokstad EL. Absorption kinetics of orally administered leucovorin calcium. *NCI Monogr.* 1987;(5):47-56.

McGuire BW, Sia LL, Leese PT, Gutierrez ML, Stokstad EL. Pharmacokinetics of leucovorin calcium after intravenous, intramuscular, and oral administration. *Clin Pharm.* 1988 Jan;7(1):52-8.

McNaught CE, Woodcock NP, Anderson AD, MacFie J. A prospective randomised trial of probiotics in critically ill patients. *Clin Nutr.* 2005 Apr;24(2):211-9.

McNaught CE, Woodcock NP, MacFie J, Mitchell CJ. A prospective randomised study of the probiotic *Lactobacillus plantarum* 299V on indices of gut barrier function in elective surgical patients. *Gut.* 2002 Dec;51(6):827-31.

Mealey BL, Rose LF. Diabetes mellitus and inflammatory periodontal diseases. *Compend Contin Educ Dent.* 2008 Sep;29(7):402-8, 410, 412-3.

Meurman JH, Stamatova I. Probiotics: contributions to oral health. *Oral Dis.* 2007 Sep;13(5):443-51.

Meyer AL, Elmadfa I, Herbacek I, Micksche M. Probiotic, as well as conventional yogurt, can enhance the stimulated production of proinflammatory cytokines. *J Hum Nutr Diet.* 2007 Dec;20(6):590-8.

Michetti P, Dorta G, Wiesel PH, Brassart D, Verdu E, Herranz M, Felley C, Porta N, Rouvet M, Blum AL, Corthésy-Theulaz I. Effect of whey-based culture supernatant of *Lactobacillus acidophilus* (johnsonii) La1 on *Helicobacter pylori* infection in humans. *Digestion.* 1999;60(3):203-9.

Michielutti F, Bertini M, Presciuttini B, Andreotti G. Clinical assessment of a new oral bacterial treatment for children with acute diarrhea. *Minerva Med.* 1996 Nov;87(11):545-50.

Milgrom P, Ly KA, Roberts MC, Rothen M, Mueller G, Yamaguchi DK. Mutans streptococci dose response to xylitol chewing gum. *J Dent Res.* 2006 Feb;85(2):177-81.

Miller JD, Morin LP, Schwartz WJ, Moore RY. New insights into the mammalian circadian clock. *Sleep.* 1996 Oct;19(8):641-67.

Modern Biology. Austin: Harcourt Brace, 1993.

Mohammad MA, Molloy A, Scott J, Hussein L. Plasma cobalamin and folate and their metabolic markers methylmalonic acid and total homocysteine among Egyptian children before and after nutritional supplementation with the probiotic bacteria *Lactobacillus acidophilus* in yoghurt matrix. *Int J Food Sci Nutr.* 2006 Nov-Dec;57(7-8):470-80.

Mohan R, Koebnick C, Schildt J, Mueller M, Radke M, Blaut M. Effects of *Bifidobacterium lactis* Bb12 supplementation on body weight, fecal pH, acetate, lactate, calprotectin, and IgA in preterm infants. *Pediatr Res.* 2008 Oct;64(4):418-22.

Mohan R, Koebnick C, Schildt J, Schmidt S, Mueller M, Possner M, Radke M, Blaut M. Effects of *Bifidobacterium lactis* Bb12 supplementation on intestinal microbiota of preterm infants: a double-blind, placebo-controlled, randomized study. *J Clin Microbiol.* 2006 Nov;44(11):4025-31.

Morimoto K, Takeshita T, Nanno M, Tokudome S, Nakayama K. Modulation of natural killer cell activity by supplementation of fermented milk containing *Lactobacillus casei* in habitual smokers. *Prev Med.* 2005 May;40(5):589-94.

Moss M. E. Coli Path Shows Flaws in Ground Beef Inspection. *NY Times* 2009 Oct 3.

Mozafar A. Is there vitamin B12 in plants or not? A plant nutritionist's view. *Veg Nutr.* 1997;1/2:50-52.

Mullié C, Yazourh A, Thibault H, Odou MF, Singer E, Kalach N, Kremp O, Romond MB. Increased poliovirus-specific intestinal antibody response coincides with promotion of *Bifidobacterium longum*-infantis and *Bifidobacterium breve* in infants: a randomized, double-blind, placebo-controlled trial. *Pediatr Res.* 2004 Nov;56(5):791-5.

Murray M and Pizzorno J. *Encyclopedia of Natural Medicine.* 2nd Edition. Roseville, CA: Prima Publishing, 1998.

Mustapha A, Jiang T, Savaiano DA. Improvement of lactose digestion by humans following ingestion of unfermented acidophilus milk: influence of bile sensitivity, lactose transport, and acid tolerance of *Lactobacillus acidophilus.* J Dairy Sci. 1997 Aug;80(8):1537-45.

Myllyluoma E, Ahonen AM, Korpela R, Vapaatalo H, Kankuri E. Effects of multispecies probiotic combination on helicobacter pylori infection in vitro. *Clin Vaccine Immunol.* 2008 Sep;15(9):1472-82.

Naito S, Koga H, Yamaguchi A, Fujimoto N, Hasui Y, Kuramoto H, Iguchi A, Kinukawa N; Kyushu University Urological Oncology Group. Prevention of recurrence with epirubicin and *Lactobacillus casei* after transurethral resection of bladder cancer. *J Urol.* 2008 Feb;179(2):485-90.

Naruszewicz M, Johansson ML, Zapolska-Downar D, Bukowska H. Effect of *Lactobacillus plantarum* 299v on cardiovascular disease risk factors in smokers. *Am J Clin Nutr.* 2002 Dec;76(6):1249-55.

Narva M, Nevala R, Poussa T, Korpela R. The effect of *Lactobacillus helveticus* fermented milk on acute changes in calcium metabolism in postmenopausal women. *Eur J Nutr.* 2004 Apr;43(2):61-8.

Näse L, Hatakka K, Savilahti E, Saxelin M, Pönkä A, Poussa T, Korpela R, Meurman JH. Effect of long-term consumption of a probiotic bacterium, *Lactobacillus rhamnosus* GG, in milk on dental caries and caries risk in children. *Caries Res.* 2001 Nov-Dec;35(6):412-20.

Nichols TC, Fischer TH, Deliargyris EN, Baldwin AS Jr. Role of nuclear factor-kappa B (NF-kappa B) in inflammation, periodontitis, and atherogenesis. *Ann Periodontol.* 2001 Dec;6(1):20-9.

Niedzielin K, Kordecki H, Birkenfeld B. A controlled, double-blind, randomized study on the efficacy of *Lactobacillus plantarum* 299V in patients with irritable bowel syndrome. *Eur J Gastroenterol Hepatol.* 2001 Oct;13(10):1143-7.

Nielsen OH, Jørgensen S, Pedersen K, Justesen T. Microbiological evaluation of jejunal aspirates and faecal samples after oral administration of bifidobacteria and lactic acid bacteria. *J Appl Bacteriol.* 1994 May;76(5):469-74.

Nilson KM, Vakil JR, Shahani KM. B-complex vitamin content of cheddar cheese. *J Nutr.* 1965 Aug;86:362-8.

Nobaek S, Johansson ML, Molin G, Ahrné S, Jeppsson B. Alteration of intestinal microflora is associated with reduction in abdominal bloating and pain in patients with irritable bowel syndrome. *Am J Gastroenterol.* 2000 May;95(5):1231-8.

Nopchinda S, Varavithya W, Phuapradit P, Sangchai R, Suthutvoravut U, Chantraruksa V, Haschke F. Effect of bifidobacterium Bb12 with or without *Streptococcus thermophilus* supplemented formula on nutritional status. *J Med Assoc Thai.* 2002 Nov;85 Suppl 4:S1225-31.

Nova E, Toro O, Varela P, López-Vidriero I, Morandé G, Marcos A. Effects of a nutritional intervention with yogurt on lymphocyte subsets and cytokine production capacity in anorexia nervosa patients. *Eur J Nutr.* 2006 Jun;45(4):225-33.

O'Brien SJ, Shannon JE, Gail MH. A molecular approach to the identification and individualization of human and animal cells in culture: isozyme and allozyme genetic signatures. *In Vitro.* 1980 Feb;16(2):119-35.

Odamaki T, Xiao JZ, Iwabuchi N, Sakamoto M, Takahashi N, Kondo S, Miyaji K, Iwatsuki K, Togashi H, Enomoto T, Benno Y. Influence of *Bifidobacterium longum* BB536 intake on faecal microbiota in individuals with Japanese cedar pollinosis during the pollen season. *J Med Microbiol.* 2007 Oct;56(Pt 10):1301-8.

Odamaki T, Xiao JZ, Iwabuchi N, Sakamoto M, Takahashi N, Kondo S, Iwatsuki K, Kokubo S, Togashi H, Enomoto T, Benno Y. Fluctuation of fecal microbiota in individuals with Japanese cedar pollinosis during the pollen season and influence of probiotic intake. *J Investig Allergol Clin Immunol.* 2007;17(2):92-100.

Ogawa T, Hashikawa S, Asai Y, Sakamoto H, Yasuda K, Makimura Y. A new synbiotic, *Lactobacillus casei* subsp. casei together with dextran, reduces murine and human allergic reaction. *FEMS Immunol Med Microbiol.* 2006 Apr;46(3):400-9.

Ohashi Y, Nakai S, Tsukamoto T, Masumori N, Akaza H, Miyanaga N, Kitamura T, Kawabe K, Kotake T, Kuroda M, Naito S, Koga H, Saito Y, Nomata K, Kitagawa M, Aso Y. Habitual intake of lactic acid bacteria and risk reduction of bladder cancer. *Urol Int*. 2002;68(4):273-80.

Okamura T, Maehara Y, Sugimachi K. Phase II clinical study of LC9018 on carcinomatous peritonitis of gastric cancer. Subgroup for Carcinomatous Peritonitis, Cooperative, Study Group of LC9018. *Gan To Kagaku Ryoho*. 1989 Jun;16(6):2257-62.

Okawa T, Niibe H, Arai T, Sekiba K, Noda K, Takeuchi S, Hashimoto S, Ogawa N. Effect of LC9018 combined with radiation therapy on carcinoma of the uterine cervix. A phase III, multicenter, randomized, controlled study. *Cancer*. 1993 Sep 15;72(6):1949-54.

Oláh A, Belágyi T, Issekutz A, Gamal ME, Bengmark S. Randomized clinical trial of specific *Lactobacillus* and fibre supplement to early enteral nutrition in patients with acute pancreatitis. *Br J Surg*. 2002 Sep;89(9):1103-7.

Oleĭnichenko EV, Mitrokhin SD, Nonikov VE, Minaev VI. Effectiveness of acipole in prevention of enteric dysbacteriosis due to antibacterial therapy. *Antibiot Khimioter*. 1999;44(1):23-5.

Olivares M, Díaz-Ropero MA, Gómez N, Lara-Villoslada F, Sierra S, Maldonado JA, Martín R, López-Huertas E, Rodríguez JM, Xaus J. Oral administration of two probiotic strains, *Lactobacillus gasseri* CECT5714 and *Lactobacillus coryniformis* CECT5711, enhances the intestinal function of healthy adults. *Int J Food Microbiol*. 2006 Mar;107(2):104-11.

Olivares M, Paz Díaz-Ropero M, Gómez N, Sierra S, Lara-Villoslada F, Martín R, Miguel Rodríguez J, Xaus J. Dietary deprivation of fermented foods causes a fall in innate immune response. Lactic acid bacteria can counteract the immunological effect of this deprivation. *J Dairy Res*. 2006 Nov;73(4):492-8.

O'Mahony L, McCarthy J, Kelly P, Hurley G, Luo F, Chen K, O'Sullivan GC, Kiely B, Collins JK, Shanahan F, Quigley EM. *Lactobacillus* and *Bifidobacterium* in irritable bowel syndrome: symptom responses and relationship to cytokine profiles. *Gastroenterology*. 2005 Mar;128(3):541-51.

Onwulata CI, Rao DR, Vankineni P. Relative efficiency of yogurt, sweet acidophilus milk, hydrolyzed-lactose milk, and a commercial lactase tablet in alleviating lactose maldigestion. *Am J Clin Nutr*. 1989 Jun;49(6):1233-7.

Oozeer R, Leplingard A, Mater DD, Mogenet A, Michelin R, Seksek I, Marteau P, Doré J, Bresson JL, Corthier G. Survival of *Lactobacillus casei* in the human digestive tract after consumption of fermented milk. *Appl Environ Microbiol*. 2006 Aug;72(8):5615-7.

Ortiz-Andrellucchi A, Sánchez-Villegas A, Rodríguez-Gallego C, Lemes A, Molero T, Soria A, Peña-Quintana L, Santana M, Ramírez O, García J, Cabrera F, Cobo J, Serra-Majem L. Immunomodulatory effects of the intake of fermented milk with *Lactobacillus casei* DN114001 in lactating mothers and their children. *Br J Nutr*. 2008 Oct;100(4):834-45.

Ouwehand AC, Bergsma N, Parhiala R, Lahtinen S, Gueimonde M, Finne-Soveri H, Strandberg T, Pitkälä K, Salminen S. *Bifidobacterium* microbiota and parameters of immune function in elderly subjects. *FEMS Immunol Med Microbiol*. 2008 Jun;53(1):18-25.

Ouwehand AC, Tiihonen K, Saarinen M, Putaala H, Rautonen N. Influence of a combination of *Lactobacillus acidophilus* NCFM and lactitol on healthy elderly: intestinal and immune parameters. *Br J Nutr*. 2009 Feb;101(3):367-75.

Ouwehand AC. Antiallergic effects of probiotics. *J Nutr*. 2007 Mar;137(3 Suppl 2):794S-7S.

Ozkan TB, Sahin E, Erdemir G, Budak F. Effect of *Saccharomyces boulardii* in children with acute gastroenteritis and its relationship to the immune response. *J Int Med Res*. 2007 Mar-Apr;35(2):201-12.

Paineau D, Carcano D, Leyer G, Darquy S, Alyanakian MA, Simoneau G, Bergmann JF, Brassart D, Bornet F, Ouwehand AC. Effects of seven potential probiotic strains on specific immune responses in healthy adults: a double-blind, randomized, controlled trial. *FEMS Immunol Med Microbiol*. 2008 Jun;53(1):107-13.

Panigrahi P, Parida S, Pradhan L, Mohapatra SS, Misra PR, Johnson JA, Chaudhry R, Taylor S, Hansen NI, Gewolb IH. Long-term colonization of a *Lactobacillus plantarum* synbiotic preparation in the neonatal gut. *J Pediatr Gastroenterol Nutr*. 2008 Jul;47(1):45-53.

Parra D, De Morentin BM, Cobo JM, Mateos A, Martinez JA. Monocyte function in healthy middle-aged people receiving fermented milk containing *Lactobacillus casei*. *J Nutr Health Aging*. 2004;8(4):208-11.

Parra MD, Martínez de Morentin BE, Cobo JM, Mateos A, Martínez JA. Daily ingestion of fermented milk containing *Lactobacillus casei* DN114001 improves innate-defense capacity in healthy middle-aged people. *J Physiol Biochem*. 2004 Jun;60(2):85-91.

Passeron T, Lacour JP, Fontas E, Ortonne JP. Prebiotics and synbiotics: two promising approaches for the treatment of atopic dermatitis in children above 2 years. *Allergy*. 2006 Apr;61(4):431-7.

Patterson DB. Anaphylactic shock from chloromycetin. Northwest Med. 1950 May;49(5):352-3. Agarwal KN, Bhasin SK. Feasibility studies to control acute diarrhoea in children by feeding fermented milk preparations Actimel and Indian Dahi. *Eur J Clin Nutr*. 2002 Dec;56 Suppl 4:S56-9.

Pedone CA, Arnaud CC, Postaire ER, Bouley CF, Reinert P. Multicentric study of the effect of milk fermented by *Lactobacillus casei* on the incidence of diarrhoea. *Int J Clin Pract.* 2000 Nov;54(9):568-71.

Pedone CA, Bernabeu AO, Postaire ER, Bouley CF, Reinert P. The effect of supplementation with milk fermented by *Lactobacillus casei* (strain DN-114 001) on acute diarrhoea in children attending day care centres. *Int J Clin Pract.* 1999 Apr-May;53(3):179-84.

Pedrosa MC, Golner BB, Goldin BR, Barakat S, Dallal GE, Russell RM. Survival of yogurt-containing organisms and *Lactobacillus gasseri* (ADH) and their effect on bacterial enzyme activity in the gastrointestinal tract of healthy and hypochlorhydric elderly subjects. *Am J Clin Nutr.* 1995 Feb;61(2):353-9.

Peral MC, Martinez MA, Valdez JC. Bacteriotherapy with *Lactobacillus plantarum* in burns. *Int Wound J.* 2009 Feb;6(1):73-81.

Persson GR, Persson RE. Cardiovascular disease and periodontitis: an update on the associations and risk. *J Clin Periodontol.* 2008 Sep;35(8 Suppl):362-79.

Persson GR. Immune responses and vaccination against periodontal infections. *J Clin Periodontol.* 2005;32 Suppl 6:39-53.

Persson R, Orbaek P, Kecklund G, Akerstedt T. Impact of an 84-hour workweek on biomarkers for stress, metabolic processes and diurnal rhythm. *Scand J Work Environ Health.* 2006 Oct;32(5):349-58.

Pessi T, Sütas Y, Hurme M, Isolauri E. Interleukin-10 generation in atopic children following oral *Lactobacillus rhamnosus* GG. *Clin Exp Allergy.* 2000 Dec;30(12):1804-8.

Petricevic L, Unger FM, Viernstein H, Kiss H. Randomized, double-blind, placebo-controlled study of oral lactobacilli to improve the vaginal flora of postmenopausal women. *Eur J Obstet Gynecol Reprod Biol.* 2008 Nov;141(1):54-7.

Petricevic L, Witt A. The role of *Lactobacillus casei* rhamnosus Lcr35 in restoring the normal vaginal flora after antibiotic treatment of bacterial vaginosis. *BJOG.* 2008 Oct;115(11):1369-74.

Petrunov B, Marinova S, Markova R, Nenkov P, Nikolaeva S, Nikolova M, Taskov H, Cvetanov J. Cellular and humoral systemic and mucosal immune responses stimulated in volunteers by an oral polybacterial immunomodulator "Dentavax". *Int Immunopharmacol.* 2006 Jul;6(7):1181-93.

Petti S, Tarsitani G, D'Arca AS. A randomized clinical trial of the effect of yoghurt on the human salivary microflora. *Arch Oral Biol.* 2001 Aug;46(8):705-12.

Phuapradit P, Varavithya W, Vathanophas K, Sangchai R, Podhipak A, Suthutvoravut U, Nopchinda S, Chantraruksa V, Haschke F. Reduction of rotavirus infection in children receiving bifidobacteria-supplemented formula. *J Med Assoc Thai.* 1999 Nov;82 Suppl 1:S43-8.

Piirainen L, Haahtela S, Helin T, Korpela R, Haahtela T, Vaarala O. Effect of *Lactobacillus rhamnosus* GG on rBet v1 and rMal d1 specific IgA in the saliva of patients with birch pollen allergy. *Ann Allergy Asthma Immunol.* 2008 Apr;100(4):338-42.

Pitkala KH, Strandberg TE, Finne Soveri UH, Ouwehand AC, Poussa T, Salminen S. Fermented cereal with specific bifidobacteria normalizes bowel movements in elderly nursing home residents. A randomized, controlled trial. *J Nutr Health Aging.* 2007 Jul-Aug;11(4):305-11.

Plein K, Hotz J. Therapeutic effects of *Saccharomyces boulardii* on mild residual symptoms in a stable phase of Crohn's disease with special respect to chronic diarrhea—a pilot study. *Z Gastroenterol.* 1993 Feb;31(2):129-34.

Pohjavuori E, Viljanen M, Korpela R, Kuitunen M, Tiittanen M, Vaarala O, Savilahti E. *Lactobacillus* GG effect in increasing IFN-gamma production in infants with cow's milk allergy. *J Allergy Clin Immunol.* 2004 Jul;114(1):131-6.

Power DA, Burton JP, Chilcott CN, Dawes PJ, Tagg JR. Preliminary investigations of the colonisation of upper respiratory tract tissues of infants using a paediatric formulation of the oral probiotic Streptococcus salivarius K12. *Eur J Clin Microbiol Infect Dis.* 2008 Dec;27(12):1261-3.

Pregliasco F, Anselmi G, Fonte L, Giussani F, Schieppati S, Soletti L. A new chance of preventing winter diseases by the administration of synbiotic formulations. *J Clin Gastroenterol.* 2008 Sep;42 Suppl 3 Pt 2:S224-33.

Prescott SL, Wickens K, Westcott L, Jung W, Currie H, Black PN, Stanley TV, Mitchell EA, Fitzharris P, Siebers R, Wu L, Crane J; Probiotic Study Group. Supplementation with *Lactobacillus rhamnosus* or *Bifidobacterium lactis* probiotics in pregnancy increases cord blood interferon-gamma and breast milk transforming growth factor-beta and immunoglobin A detection. *Clin Exp Allergy.* 2008 Oct;38(10):1606-14.

Qin HL, Zheng JJ, Tong DN, Chen WX, Fan XB, Hang XM, Jiang YQ. Effect of *Lactobacillus plantarum* enteral feeding on the gut permeability and septic complications in the patients with acute pancreatitis. *Eur J Clin Nutr.* 2008 Jul;62(7):923-30.

Rafter J, Bennett M, Caderni G, Clune Y, Hughes R, Karlsson PC, Klinder A, O'Riordan M, O'Sullivan GC, Pool-Zobel B, Rechkemmer G, Roller M, Rowland I, Salvadori M, Thijs H, Van Loo J, Watzl B, Collins JK. Dietary synbiotics reduce cancer risk factors in polypectomized and colon cancer patients. *Am J Clin Nutr.* 2007 Feb;85(2):488-96.

Randal Bollinger R, Barbas AS, Bush EL, Lin SS, Parker W. Biofilms in the large bowel suggest an apparent function of the human vermiform appendix. *J Theor Biol.* 2007 Dec 21;249(4):826-31.

Rangavajhyala N, Shahani KM, Sridevi G, Srikumaran S. Nonlipopolysaccharide component(s) of *Lactobacillus acidophilus* stimulate(s) the production of interleukin-1 alpha and tumor necrosis factor-alpha by murine macrophages. *Nutr Cancer.* 1997;28(2):130-4.

Rautava S, Salminen S, Isolauri E. Specific probiotics in reducing the risk of acute infections in infancy—a randomised, double-blind, placebo-controlled study. *Br J Nutr.* 2009 Jun;101(11):1722-6.

Rayes N, Seehofer D, Hansen S, Boucsein K, Müller AR, Serke S, Bengmark S, Neuhaus P. Early enteral supply of lactobacillus and fiber versus selective bowel decontamination: a controlled trial in liver transplant recipients. *Transplantation.* 2002 Jul 15;74(1):123-7.

Rayes N, Seehofer D, Müller AR, Hansen S, Bengmark S, Neuhaus P. Influence of probiotics and fibre on the incidence of bacterial infections following major abdominal surgery - results of a prospective trial. *Z Gastroenterol.* 2002 Oct;40(10):869-76.

Raza S, Graham SM, Allen SJ, Sultana S, Cuevas L, Hart CA, Kaila M, Isolauri E, Saxelin M, Arvilommi H, *et al. Lactobacillus* GG in acute diarrhea. *Indian Pediatr.* 1995 Oct;32(10):1140-2.

Raza S, Graham SM, Allen SJ, Sultana S, Cuevas L, Hart CA. *Lactobacillus* GG promotes recovery from acute nonbloody diarrhea in Pakistan. Pediatr Infect Dis J. 1995 Feb;14(2):107-11.

Reddy KP, Shahani KM, Kulkarni SM. B-complex vitamins in cultured and acidified yogurt. *J Dairy Sci.* 1976 Feb;59(2):191-5.

Reger D, Goode S, Mercer E. *Chemistry: Principles & Practice.* Fort Worth, TX: Harcourt Brace, 1993.

Regis E. *Virus Ground Zero.* New York: Pocket, 1996.

Reid G, Beuerman D, Heinemann C, Bruce AW. Probiotic *Lactobacillus* dose required to restore and maintain a normal vaginal flora. *FEMS Immunol Med Microbiol.* 2001 Dec;32(1):37-41.

Reid G, Burton J, Hammond JA, Bruce AW. Nucleic acid-based diagnosis of bacterial vaginosis and improved management using probiotic lactobacilli. *J Med Food.* 2004 Summer;7(2):223-8.

Reid G, Charbonneau D, Erb J, Kochanowski B, Beuerman D, Poehner R, Bruce AW. Oral use of *Lactobacillus rhamnosus* GR-1 and L. fermentum RC-14 significantly alters vaginal flora: randomized, placebo-controlled trial in 64 healthy women. *FEMS Immunol Med Microbiol.* 2003 Mar 20;35(2):131-4.

Renvert S, Lindahl C, Renvert H, Persson GR. Clinical and microbiological analysis of subjects treated with Brånemark or AstraTech implants: a 7-year follow-up study. *Clin Oral Implants Res.* 2008 Apr;19(4):342-7.

Riccia DN, Bizzini F, Perilli MG, Polimeni A, Trinchieri V, Amicosante G, Cifone MG. Anti-inflammatory effects of *Lactobacillus brevis* (CD2) on periodontal disease. *Oral Dis.* 2007 Jul;13(4):376-85.

Rinne M, Kalliomaki M, Arvilommi H, Salminen S, Isolauri E. Effect of probiotics and breastfeeding on the bifidobacterium and lactobacillus/enterococcus microbiota and humoral immune responses. *J Pediatr.* 2005 Aug;147(2):186-91.

Rinne M, Kalliomäki M, Salminen S, Isolauri E. Probiotic intervention in the first months of life: short-term effects on gastrointestinal symptoms and long-term effects on gut microbiota. *J Pediatr Gastroenterol Nutr.* 2006 Aug;43(2):200-5.

Río ME, Zago Beatriz L, Garcia H, Winter L. The nutritional status change the effectiveness of a dietary supplement of lactic bacteria on the emerging of respiratory tract diseases in children. *Arch Latinoam Nutr.* 2002 Mar;52(1):29-34.

Río ME, Zago LB, Garcia H, Winter L. Influence of nutritional status on the effectiveness of a dietary supplement of live lactobacillus to prevent and cure diarrhoea in children. *Arch Latinoam Nutr.* 2004 Sep;54(3):287-92.

Roessler A, Friedrich U, Vogelsang H, Bauer A, Kaatz M, Hipler UC, Schmidt I, Jahreis G. The immune system in healthy adults and patients with atopic dermatitis seems to be affected differently by a probiotic intervention. *Clin Exp Allergy.* 2008 Jan;38(1):93-102.

Roller M, Clune Y, Collins K, Rechkemmer G, Watzl B. Consumption of prebiotic inulin enriched with oligofructose in combination with the probiotics *Lactobacillus rhamnosus* and *Bifidobacterium lactis* has minor effects on selected immune parameters in polypectomised and colon cancer patients. *Br J Nutr.* 2007 Apr;97(4):676-84.

Rosander A, Connolly E, Roos S. Removal of antibiotic resistance gene-carrying plasmids from *Lactobacillus reuteri* ATCC 55730 and characterization of the resulting daughter strain, L. reuteri DSM 17938. *Appl Environ Microbiol.* 2008 Oct;74(19):6032-40.

Rosenfeldt V, Benfeldt E, Valerius NH, Paerregaard A, Michaelsen KF. Effect of probiotics on gastrointestinal symptoms and small intestinal permeability in children with atopic dermatitis. *J Pediatr.* 2004 Nov;145(5):612-6.

Rousseaux C, Thuru X, Gelot A, Barnich N, Neut C, Dubuquoy L, Dubuquoy C, Merour E, Geboes K, Chamaillard M, Ouwehand A, Leyer G, Carcano D, Colombel JF, Ardid D, Desreumaux P. *Lactobacil-*

REFERENCES AND BIBLIOGRAPHY

lus acidophilus modulates intestinal pain and induces opioid and cannabinoid receptors. *Nat Med.* 2007 Jan;13(1):35-7

Saavedra JM, Abi-Hanna A, Moore N, Yolken RH. Long-term consumption of infant formulas containing live probiotic bacteria: tolerance and safety. *Am J Clin Nutr.* 2004 Feb;79(2):261-7.

Saavedra JM, Bauman NA, Oung I, Perman JA, Yolken RH. Feeding of *Bifidobacterium bifidum* and *Streptococcus thermophilus* to infants in hospital for prevention of diarrhoea and shedding of rotavirus. *Lancet.* 1994 Oct 15;344(8929):1046-9.

Saggioro A. Probiotics in the treatment of irritable bowel syndrome. *J Clin Gastroenterol.* 2004 Jul;38(6 Suppl):S104-6.

Sahagún-Flores JE, López-Peña LS, de la Cruz-Ramírez Jaimes J, García-Bravo MS, Peregrina-Gómez R, de Alba-García JE. Eradication of *Helicobacter pylori*: triple treatment scheme plus *Lactobacillus* vs. triple treatment alone. *Cir Cir.* 2007 Sep-Oct;75(5):333-6.

Salazar-Lindo E, Figueroa-Quintanilla D, Caciano MI, Reto-Valiente V, Chauviere G, Colin P; Lacteol Study Group. Effectiveness and safety of *Lactobacillus* LB in the treatment of mild acute diarrhea in children. *J Pediatr Gastroenterol Nutr.* 2007 May;44(5):571-6.

Salazar-Lindo E, Miranda-Langschwager P, Campos-Sanchez M, Chea-Woo E, Sack RB. *Lactobacillus casei* strain GG in the treatment of infants with acute watery diarrhea: a randomized, double-blind, placebo controlled clinical trial [ISRCTN67363048]. *BMC Pediatr.* 2004 Sep 2;4:18.

Salminen E, Elomaa I, Minkkinen J, Vapaatalo H, Salminen S. Preservation of intestinal integrity during radiotherapy using live *Lactobacillus acidophilus* cultures. *Clin Radiol.* 1988 Jul;39(4):435-7.

Samanta M, Sarkar M, Ghosh P, Ghosh J, Sinha M, Chatterjee S. Prophylactic probiotics for prevention of necrotizing enterocolitis in very low birth weight newborns. *J Trop Pediatr.* 2009 Apr;55(2):128-31.

Saran S, Gopalan S, Krishna TP. Use of fermented foods to combat stunting and failure to thrive. *Nutrition.* 2002 May;18(5):393-6.

Savino F, Pelle E, Palumeri E, Oggero R, Miniero R. *Lactobacillus reuteri* (American Type Culture Collection Strain 55730) versus simethicone in the treatment of infantile colic: a prospective randomized study. *Pediatrics.* 2007 Jan;119(1):e124-30.

Schaafsma G, Meuling WJ, van Dokkum W, Bouley C. Effects of a milk product, fermented by *Lactobacillus acidophilus* and with fructo-oligosaccharides added, on blood lipids in male volunteers. *Eur J Clin Nutr.* 1998 Jun;52(6):436-40.

Schiffrin EJ, Brassart D, Servin AL, Rochat F, Donnet-Hughes A. Immune modulation of blood leukocytes in humans by lactic acid bacteria: criteria for strain selection. *Am J Clin Nutr.* 1997 Aug;66(2):515S-520S.

Scholz-Ahrens KE, Ade P, Marten B, Weber P, Timm W, Açil Y, Glüer CC, Schrezenmeir J. Prebiotics, probiotics, and synbiotics affect mineral absorption, bone mineral content, and bone structure. *J Nutr.* 2007 Mar;137(3 Suppl 2):838S-46S.

Schulman G. A nexus of progression of chronic kidney disease: charcoal, tryptophan and profibrotic cytokines. *Blood Purif.* 2006;24(1):143-8.

Schumacher P. *Biophysical Therapy Of Allergies.* Stuttgart: Thieme, 2005.

Sekine K, Toida T, Saito M, Kuboyama M, Kawashima T, Hashimoto Y. A new morphologically characterized cell wall preparation (whole peptidoglycan) from *Bifidobacterium* infantis with a higher efficacy on the regression of an established tumor in mice. *Cancer Res.* 1985 Mar;45(3):1300-7.

Seppo L, Jauhiainen T, Poussa T, Korpela R. A fermented milk high in bioactive peptides has a blood pressure-lowering effect in hypertensive subjects. *Am J Clin Nutr.* 2003 Feb;77(2):326-30.

Shahani KM, Ayebo AD. Role of dietary lactobacilli in gastrointestinal microecology. *Am J Clin Nutr.* 1980 Nov;33(11 Suppl):2448-57.

Shahani KM, Chandan RC. Nutritional and healthful aspects of cultured and culture-containing dairy foods. *J Dairy Sci.* 1979 Oct;62(10):1685-94.

Shahani KM, Friend BA. Properties of and prospects for cultured dairy foods. *Soc Appl Bacteriol Symp Ser.* 1983;11:257-69.

Shahani KM, Herper WJ, Jensen RG, Parry RM Jr, Zittle CA. Enzymes in bovine milk: a review. *J Dairy Sci.* 1973 May;56(5):531-43.

Shahani KM, Kwan AJ, Friend BA. Role and significance of enzymes in human milk. *Am J Clin Nutr.* 1980 Aug;33(8):1861-8.

Shahani KM, Meshbesher BF, Mangalampalli V. *Cultivate Health From Within.* Vital Health Publ: Danbury, CT, 2005.

Shalev E, Battino S, Weiner E, Colodner R, Keness Y. Ingestion of yogurt containing *Lactobacillus acidophilus* compared with pasteurized yogurt as prophylaxis for recurrent *Candidal* vaginitis and bacterial vaginosis. *Arch Fam Med.* 1996 Nov-Dec;5(10):593-6.

Shamir R, Makhoul IR, Etzioni A, Shehadeh N. Evaluation of a diet containing probiotics and zinc for the treatment of mild diarrheal illness in children younger than one year of age. *J Am Coll Nutr.* 2005 Oct;24(5):370-5.

Sharma P, Sharma BC, Puri V, Sarin SK. An open-label randomized controlled trial of lactulose and probiotics in the treatment of minimal hepatic encephalopathy. *Eur J Gastroent Hepatol.* 2008 Jun;20(6):506-11.

Sheih YH, Chiang BL, Wang LH, Liao CK, Gill HS. Systemic immunity-enhancing effects in healthy subjects following dietary consumption of the lactic acid bacterium *Lactobacillus rhamnosus* HN001. *J Am Coll Nutr.* 2001 Apr;20(2 Suppl):149-56.

Shimauchi H, Mayanagi G, Nakaya S, Minamibuchi M, Ito Y, Yamaki K, Hirata H. Improvement of periodontal condition by probiotics with *Lactobacillus salivarius* WB21: a randomized, double-blind, placebo-controlled study. *J Clin Periodontol.* 2008 Oct;35(10):897-905.

Shimizu K, Ogura H, Goto M, Asahara T, Nomoto K, Morotomi M, Matsushima A, Tasaki O, Fujita K, Hosotsubo H, Kuwagata Y, Tanaka H, Shimazu T, Sugimoto H. Synbiotics decrease the incidence of septic complications in patients with severe SIRS: a preliminary report. *Dig Dis Sci.* 2009 May;54(5):1071-8.

Shoaf K, Mulvey GL, Armstrong GD, Hutkins RW. Prebiotic galactooligosaccharides reduce adherence of enteropathogenic *Escherichia coli* to tissue culture cells. Infect Immun. 2006 Dec;74(12):6920-8.

Shornikova AV, Casas IA, Isolauri E, Mykkänen E, Vesikari T. *Lactobacillus reuteri* as a therapeutic agent in acute diarrhea in young children. *J Pediatr Gastroenterol Nutr.* 1997 Apr;24(4):399-404.

Shornikova AV, Casas IA, Mykkänen H, Salo E, Vesikari T. Bacteriotherapy with *Lactobacillus reuteri* in rotavirus gastroenteritis. *Pediatr Infect Dis J.* 1997 Dec;16(12):1103-7.

Silva MR, Dias G, Ferreira CL, Franceschini SC, Costa NM. Growth of preschool children was improved when fed an iron-fortified fermented milk beverage supplemented with *Lactobacillus acidophilus*. *Nutr Res.* 2008 Apr;28(4):226-32.

Simakachorn N, Pichaipat V, Rithipornpaisarn P, Kongkaew C, Tongpradit P, Varavithya W. Clinical evaluation of the addition of lyophilized, heat-killed *Lactobacillus acidophilus* LB to oral rehydration therapy in the treatment of acute diarrhea in children. *J Pediatr Gastroenterol Nutr.* 2000 Jan;30(1):68-72.

Simenhoff ML, Dunn SR, Zollner GP, Fitzpatrick ME, Emery SM, Sandine WE, Ayres JW. Biomodulation of the toxic and nutritional effects of small bowel bacterial overgrowth in end-stage kidney disease using freeze-dried *Lactobacillus acidophilus*. *Miner Electrolyte Metab.* 1996;22(1-3):92-6.

Sinn DH, Song JH, Kim HJ, Lee JH, Son HJ, Chang DK, Kim YH, Kim JJ, Rhee JC, Rhee PL. Therapeutic effect of *Lactobacillus acidophilus*-SDC 2012, 2013 in patients with irritable bowel syndrome. *Dig Dis Sci.* 2008 Oct;53(10):2714-8.

Sistek D, Kelly R, Wickens K, Stanley T, Fitzharris P, Crane J. Is the effect of probiotics on atopic dermatitis confined to food sensitized children? *Clin Exp Allergy.* 2006 May;36(5):629-33.

Skovbjerg S, Roos K, Holm SE, Grahn Håkansson E, Nowrouzian F, Ivarsson M, Adlerberth I, Wold AE. Spray bacteriotherapy decreases middle ear fluid in children with secretory otitis media. *Arch Dis Child.* 2009 Feb;94(2):92-8.

Solomons NW, Guerrero AM, Torun B. Effective in vivo hydrolysis of milk lactose by beta-galactosidases in the presence of solid foods. *Am J Clin Nutr.* 1985 Feb;41(2):222-7.

Stadlbauer V, Mookerjee RP, Hodges S, Wright GA, Davies NA, Jalan R. Effect of probiotic treatment on deranged neutrophil function and cytokine responses in patients with compensated alcoholic cirrhosis. *J Hepatol.* 2008 Jun;48(6):945-51.

Stratiki Z, Costalos C, Sevastiadou S, Kastanidou O, Skouroliakou M, Giakoumatou A, Petrohilou V. The effect of a bifidobacter supplemented bovine milk on intestinal permeability of preterm infants. *Early Hum Dev.* 2007 Sep;83(9):575-9.

Strozzi GP, Mogna L. Quantification of folic acid in human feces after administration of *Bifidobacterium* probiotic strains. *J Clin Gastroenterol.* 2008 Sep;42 Suppl 3 Pt 2:S179-84.

Sturtzel B, Mikulits C, Gisinger C, Elmadfa I. Use of fiber instead of laxative treatment in a geriatric hospital to improve the wellbeing of seniors. *J Nutr Health Aging.* 2009 Feb;13(2):136-9.

Su P, Henriksson A, Tandianus JE, Park JH, Foong F, Dunn NW. Detection and quantification of *Bifidobacterium lactis* LAFTI B94 in human faecal samples from a consumption trial. *FEMS Microbiol Lett.* 2005 Mar 1;244(1):99-103.

Sugawara G, Nagino M, Nishio H, Ebata T, Takagi K, Asahara T, Nomoto K, Nimura Y. Perioperative synbiotic treatment to prevent postoperative infectious complications in biliary cancer surgery: a randomized controlled trial. *Ann Surg.* 2006 Nov;244(5):706-14.

Sullivan A, Barkholt L, Nord CE. *Lactobacillus acidophilus*, *Bifidobacterium lactis* and *Lactobacillus* F19 prevent antibiotic-associated ecological disturbances of Bacteroides fragilis in the intestine. *J Antimicrob Chemother.* 2003 Aug;52(2):308-11.

REFERENCES AND BIBLIOGRAPHY

Szymański H, Chmielarczyk A, Strus M, Pejcz J, Jawień M, Kochan P, Heczko PB. Colonisation of the gastrointestinal tract by probiotic *L. rhamnosus* strains in acute diarrhoea in children. *Dig Liver Dis.* 2006 Dec;38 Suppl 2:S274-6.

Szymański H, Pejcz J, Jawień M, Chmielarczyk A, Strus M, Heczko PB. Treatment of acute infectious diarrhoea in infants and children with a mixture of three *Lactobacillus rhamnosus* strains—a randomized, double-blind, placebo-controlled trial. *Aliment Pharmacol Ther.* 2006 Jan 15;23(2):247-53.

Tagg JR. Prevention of streptococcal pharyngitis by anti-Streptococcus pyogenes bacteriocin-like inhibitory substances (BLIS) produced by Streptococcus salivarius. *Indian J Med Res.* 2004 May;119 Suppl:13-6.

Takagi A, Ikemura H, Matsuzaki T, Sato M, Nomoto K, Morotomi M, Yokokura T. Relationship between the in vitro response of dendritic cells to *Lactobacillus* and prevention of tumorigenesis in the mouse. *J Gastroenterol.* 2008;43(9):661-9.

Takeda K, Okumura K. Effects of a fermented milk drink containing *Lactobacillus casei* strain Shirota on the human NK-cell activity. *J Nutr.* 2007 Mar;137(3 Suppl 2):791S-3S.

Takeda K, Suzuki T, Shimada SI, Shida K, Nanno M, Okumura K. Interleukin-12 is involved in the enhancement of human natural killer cell activity by *Lactobacillus casei* Shirota. *Clin Exp Immunol.* 2006 Oct;146(1):109-15.

Tamura M, Shikina T, Morihana T, Hayama M, Kajimoto O, Sakamoto A, Kajimoto Y, Watanabe O, Nonaka C, Shida K, Nanno M. Effects of probiotics on allergic rhinitis induced by Japanese cedar pollen: randomized double-blind, placebo-controlled clinical trial. *Int Arch Allergy Imml.* 2007;143(1):75-82.

Tasli L, Mat C, De Simone C, Yazici H. Lactobacilli lozenges in the management of oral ulcers of Behçet's syndrome. *Clin Exp Rheumatol.* 2006 Sep-Oct;24(5 Suppl 42):S83-6.

Teitelbaum J. *From Fatigue to Fantastic.* New York: Avery, 2001.

Tevini M, ed. *UV-B Radiation and Ozone Depletion: Effects on humans, animals, plants, microorganisms and materials.* Boca Raton: Lewis Pub, 1993.

Thibault H, Aubert-Jacquin C, Goulet O. Effects of long-term consumption of a fermented infant formula (with *Bifidobacterium breve* c50 and *Streptococcus thermophilus* 065) on acute diarrhea in healthy infants. *J Pediatr Gastroenterol Nutr.* 2004 Aug;39(2):147-52.

Thomas Y, Schiff M, Belkadi L, Jurgens P, Kahhak L, Benveniste J. Activation of human neutrophils by electronically transmitted phorbol-myristate acetate. *Med Hypoth.* 2000;54: 33-39.

Thompson D. *On Growth and Form.* Cambridge: Cambridge University Press, 1992.

Tietze H. *Kombucha: The Miracle Fungus.* Gateway Books: Bath, UK, 1995.

Tlaskalová-Hogenová H, Stepánková R, Hudcovic T, Tucková L, Cukrowska B, Lodinová-Zádníková R, Kozáková H, Rossmann P, Bártová J, Sokol D, Funda DP, Borovská D, Reháková Z, Sinkora J, Hofman J, Drastich P, Kokesová A. Commensal bacteria (normal microflora), mucosal immunity and chronic inflammatory and autoimmune diseases. *Immunol Lett.* 2004 May 15;93(2-3):97-108.

Tormo Carnicer R, Infante Piña D, Roselló Mayans E, Bartolomé Comas R. Intake of fermented milk containing *Lactobacillus casei* DN-114 001 and its effect on gut flora. *An Pediatr.* 2006 Nov;65(5):448-53.

Touhami M, Boudraa G, Mary JY, Soltana R, Desjeux JF. Clinical consequences of replacing milk with yogurt in persistent infantile diarrhea. *Ann Pediatr.* 1992 Feb;39(2):79-86.

Trenev N. *Probiotics: Nature's Internal Healers.* New York: Avery, 1998.

Trois L, Cardoso EM, Miura E. Use of probiotics in HIV-infected children: a randomized double-blind controlled study. *J Trop Pediatr.* 2008 Feb;54(1):19-24.

Tsuchiya J, Barreto R, Okura R, Kawakita S, Fesce E, Marotta F. Single-blind follow-up study on the effectiveness of a symbiotic preparation in irritable bowel syndrome. *Chin J Dig Dis.* 2004;5(4):169-74.

Tubelius P, Stan V, Zachrisson A. Increasing work-place healthiness with the probiotic *Lactobacillus reuteri*: a randomised, double-blind placebo-controlled study. *Environ Health.* 2005 Nov 7;4:25.

Tuomilehto J, Lindström J, Hyyrynen J, Korpela R, Karhunen ML, Mikkola L, Jauhiainen T, Seppo L, Nissinen A. Effect of ingesting sour milk fermented using *Lactobacillus helveticus* bacteria producing tripeptides on blood pressure in subjects with mild hypertension. *J Hum Hypertens.* 2004 Nov;18(11):795-802.

Turchet P, Laurenzano M, Auboiron S, Antoine JM. Effect of fermented milk containing the probiotic *Lactobacillus casei* DN-114001 on winter infections in free-living elderly subjects: a randomised, controlled pilot study. *J Nutr Health Aging.* 2003;7(2):75-7.

Tursi A, Brandimarte G, Giorgetti GM, Elisei W. Mesalazine and/or *Lactobacillus casei* in maintaining long-term remission of symptomatic uncomplicated diverticular disease of the colon. *Hepatogastroenterology.* 2008 May-Jun;55(84):916-20.

Twetman S, Derawi B, Keller M, Ekstrand K, Yucel-Lindberg T, Stecksen-Blicks C. Short-term effect of chewing gums containing probiotic *Lactobacillus reuteri* on the levels of inflammatory mediators in gingival crevicular fluid. *Acta Odontol Scand.* 2009 Feb;67(1):19-24.

Unknown. Proteolytic activity of various lactic acid bacteria. *Japan Jnl Dairy Food Sci.* 1990;39(4).

Vakil JR, Shahani KM. Carbohydrate metabolism of lactic acid cultures. V. Lactobionate and gluconate metabolism of *Streptococcus lactis* UN. *J Dairy Sci.* 1969 Dec;52(12):1928-34.

Valeur N, Engel P, Carbajal N, Connolly E, Ladefoged K. Colonization and immunomodulation by *Lactobacillus reuteri* ATCC 55730 in the human gastrointestinal tract. *Appl Environ Microbiol.* 2004 Feb;70(2):1176-81.

van Baarlen P, Troost FJ, van Hemert S, van der Meer C, de Vos WM, de Groot PJ, Hooiveld GJ, Brummer RJ, Kleerebezem M. Differential NF-kappaB pathways induction by *Lactobacillus plantarum* in the duodenum of healthy humans correlating with immune tolerance. *Proc Natl Acad Sci U S A.* 2009 Feb 17;106(7):2371-6

van den Heuvel EG, Schoterman MH, Muijs T. Transgalactooligosaccharides stimulate calcium absorption in postmenopausal women. *J Nutr.* 2000 Dec;130(12):2938-42.

Vendt N, Grünberg H, Tuure T, Malminiemi O, Wuolijoki E, Tillmann V, Sepp E, Korpela R. Growth during the first 6 months of life in infants using formula enriched with *Lactobacillus rhamnosus* GG: double-blind, randomized trial. *J Hum Nutr Diet.* 2006 Feb;19(1):51-8.

Venturi A, Gionchetti P, Rizzello F, Johansson R, Zucconi E, Brigidi P, Matteuzzi D, Campieri M. Impact on the composition of the faecal flora by a new probiotic preparation: preliminary data on maintenance treatment of patients with ulcerative colitis. *Aliment Pharmacol Ther.* 1999 Aug;13(8):1103-8.

Villarruel G, Rubio DM, Lopez F, Cintioni J, Gurevech R, Romero G, Vandenplas Y. *Saccharomyces boulardii* in acute childhood diarrhoea: a randomized, placebo-controlled study. *Acta Paediatr.* 2007 Apr;96(4):538-41.

Vivatvakin B, Kowitdamrong E. Randomized control trial of live *Lactobacillus acidophilus* plus *Bifidobacterium infantis* in treatment of infantile acute watery diarrhea. *J Med Assoc Thai.* 2006 Sep;89 Suppl 3:S126-33.

Wang KY, Li SN, Liu CS, Perng DS, Su YC, Wu DC, Jan CM, Lai CH, Wang TN, Wang WM. Effects of ingesting *Lactobacillus-* and *Bifidobacterium-*containing yogurt in subjects with colonized *Helicobacter pylori. Am J Clin Nutr.* 2004 Sep;80(3):737-41.

Washio J, Sato T, Koseki T, Takahashi N. Hydrogen sulfide-producing bacteria in tongue biofilm and their relationship with oral malodour. *J Med Microbiol.* 2005 Sep;54(Pt 9):889-95.

Watson L. *Supernature.* New York: Bantam, 1973.

Watve MG, Tickoo R, Jog MM, Bhole BD. How many antibiotics are produced by the genus Streptomyces? *Arch Microbiol.* 2001 Nov;176(5):386-90.

Weekes DJ. Management of Herpes Simplex with Virostatic Bacterial Agent. *EENT Dig.* 1963;25(12).

Weekes DJ. The treatment of aphthous stomatitis with *Lactobacillus* tablets. *NY State J Med.* 1958 Aug 15;58(16):2672-3.

Weizman Z, Asli G, Alsheikh A. Effect of a probiotic infant formula on infections in child care centers: comparison of two probiotic agents. *Pediatrics.* 2005 Jan;115(1):5-9.

Wenus C, Goll R, Loken EB, Biong AS, Halvorsen DS, Florholmen J. Prevention of antibiotic-associated diarrhoea by a fermented probiotic milk drink. *Eur J Clin Nutr.* 2008 Feb;62(2):299-301.

Wescombe PA, Burton JP, Cadieux PA, Klesse NA, Hyink O, Heng NC, Chilcott CN, Reid G, Tagg JR. Megaplasmids encode differing combinations of lantibiotics in Streptococcus salivarius. *Antonie Van Leeuwenhoek.* 2006 Oct;90(3):269-80.

Wescombe PA, Upton M, Dierksen KP, Ragland NL, Sivabalan S, Wirawan RE, Inglis MA, Moore CJ, Walker GV, Chilcott CN, Jenkinson HF, Tagg JR. Production of the lantibiotic salivaricin A and its variants by oral streptococci and use of a specific induction assay to detect their presence in human saliva. *Appl Environ Microbiol.* 2006 Feb;72(2):1459-66.

West R. Risk of death in meat and non-meat eaters. *BMJ.* 1994 Oct 8;309(6959):955.

Wheeler JG, Bogle ML, Shema SJ, Shirrell MA, Stine KC, Pittler AJ, Burks AW, Helm RM. Impact of dietary yogurt on immune function. *Am J Med Sci.* 1997 Feb;313(2):120-3.

Wheeler JG, Shema SJ, Bogle ML, Shirrell MA, Burks AW, Pittler A, Helm RM. Immune and clinical impact of *Lactobacillus acidophilus* on asthma. *Ann Allergy Asthma Immunol.* 1997 Sep;79(3):229-33.

Whorwell PJ, Altringer L, Morel J, Bond Y, Charbonneau D, O'Mahony L, Kiely B, Shanahan F, Quigley EM. Efficacy of an encapsulated probiotic *Bifidobacterium infantis* 35624 in women with irritable bowel syndrome. *Am J Gastroenterol.* 2006 Jul;101(7):1581-90.

Wickens K, Black PN, Stanley TV, Mitchell E, Fitzharris P, Tannock GW, Purdie G, Crane J; Probiotic Study Group. A differential effect of 2 probiotics in the prevention of eczema and atopy: a double-blind, randomized, placebo-controlled trial. *J Allergy Clin Immunol.* 2008 Oct;122(4):788-94.

Wildt S, Munck LK, Vinter-Jensen L, Hanse BF, Nordgaard-Lassen I, Christensen S, Avnstroem S, Rasmussen SN, Rumessen JJ. Probiotic treatment of collagenous colitis: a randomized, double-blind, placebo-controlled trial with *Lactobacillus acidophilus* and *Bifidobacterium animalis* subsp. *Lactis. Inflamm Bowel Dis.* 2006 May;12(5):395-401.

Williams AB, Yu C, Tashima K, Burgess J, Danvers K. Evaluation of two self-care treatments for prevention of vaginal candidiasis in women with HIV. *J Assoc Nurses AIDS Care.* 2001 Jul-Aug;12(4):51-7.

Witsell DL, Garrett CG, Yarbrough WG, Dorrestein SP, Drake AF, Weissler MC. Effect of *Lactobacillus acidophilus* on antibiotic-associated gastrointestinal morbidity: a prospective randomized trial. *J Otolaryngol.* 1995 Aug;24(4):230-3.

Wu Q, Wu K, Ye Y, Dong X, Zhang J. Quorum sensing and its roles in pathogenesis among animal-associated pathogens—a review. *Wei Sheng Wu Xue Bao.* 2009 Jul 4;49(7):853-8.

Xiao JZ, Kondo S, Takahashi N, Miyaji K, Oshida K, Hiramatsu A, Iwatsuki K, Kokubo S, Hosono A. Effects of milk products fermented by *Bifidobacterium longum* on blood lipids in rats and healthy adult male volunteers. *J Dairy Sci.* 2003 Jul;86(7):2452-61.

Xiao JZ, Kondo S, Yanagisawa N, Miyaji K, Enomoto K, Sakoda T, Iwatsuki K, Enomoto T. Clinical efficacy of probiotic *Bifidobacterium longum* for the treatment of symptoms of Japanese cedar pollen allergy in subjects evaluated in an environmental exposure unit. *Allergol Int.* 2007 Mar;56(1):67-75.

Xiao JZ, Kondo S, Yanagisawa N, Takahashi N, Odamaki T, Iwabuchi N, Miyaji K, Iwatsuki K, Togashi H, Enomoto K, Enomoto T. Probiotics in the treatment of Japanese cedar pollinosis: a double-blind placebo-controlled trial. *Clin Exp Allergy.* 2006 Nov;36(11):1425-35.

Xiao JZ, Kondo S, Yanagisawa N, Takahashi N, Odamaki T, Iwabuchi N, Iwatsuki K, Kokubo S, Togashi H, Enomoto K, Enomoto T. Effect of probiotic *Bifidobacterium longum* BB536 in relieving clinical symptoms and modulating plasma cytokine levels of Japanese cedar pollinosis during the pollen season. A randomized double-blind, placebo-controlled trial. *J Investig Allergol Clin Immunol.* 2006;16(2):86-93.

Xiao SD, Zhang DZ, Lu H, Jiang SH, Liu HY, Wang GS, Xu GM, Zhang ZB, Lin GJ, Wang GL. Multicenter, randomized, controlled trial of heat-killed *Lactobacillus acidophilus* LB in patients with chronic diarrhea. *Adv Ther.* 2003 Sep-Oct;20(5):253-60.

Yadav H, Jain S, Sinha PR. Antidiabetic effect of probiotic dahl containing *Lactobacillus acidophilus* and *Lactobacillus casei* in high fructose fed rats. *Nutrition.* 2007 Jan;23(1):62-8.

Yamamura S, Morishima H, Kumano-go T, Suganuma N, Matsumoto H, Adachi H, Sigedo Y, Mikami A, Kai T, Masuyama A, Takano T, Sugita Y, Takeda M. The effect of *Lactobacillus helveticus* fermented milk on sleep and health perception in elderly subjects. *Eur J Clin Nutr.* 2009 Jan;63(1):100-5.

Yamauchi S, Ikeda M, Ikeda M, Yoshida A, Okamoto K, Ozawa A. Immunological Considerations in patients with tonsillar lesions. *Tokai J Exp Clin Med.* 1981 Apr;6(2):181-92.

Yasuda T, Takeyama Y, Ueda T, Shinzeki M, Sawa H, Nakajima T, Kuroda Y. Breakdown of Intestinal Mucosa Via Accelerated Apoptosis Increases Intestinal Permeability in Experimental Severe Acute Pancreatitis. *J Surg Res.* 2006 Apr 4.

Yeager S. The Doctor's Book of Food Remedies. Emmaus, PA: Rodale Press, 1998.

Zahradnik RT, Magnusson I, Walker C, McDonell E, Hillman CH, Hillman JD. Preliminary assessment of safety and effectiveness in humans of ProBiora3, a probiotic mouthwash. *J Appl Microbiol.* 2009 Aug;107(2):682-90.

Zarate G, Gonzalez S, Chaia AP. *Assessing survival of dairy propionibacteria in gastrointestinal conditions and adherence to intestinal epithelia. Centro de Referencia para Lactobacilos-CONICET.* Tucuman, Argentina: Humana Press. 2004.

Zeng J, Li YQ, Zuo XL, Zhen YB, Yang J, Liu CH. Clinical trial: effect of active lactic acid bacteria on mucosal barrier function in patients with diarrhoea-predominant irritable bowel syndrome. *Aliment Pharmacol Ther.* 2008 Oct 15;28(8):994-1002.

Zhao HY, Wang HJ, Lu Z, Xu SZ. Intestinal microflora in patients with liver cirrhosis. *Chin J Dig Dis.* 2004;5(2):64-7.

Ziemniak W. Efficacy of *Helicobacter pylori* eradication taking into account its resistance to antibiotics. *J Physiol Pharmacol.* 2006 Sep;57 Suppl 3:123-41.

Zwolińska-Wcisło M, Brzozowski T, Mach T, Budak A, Trojanowska D, Konturek PC, Pajdo R, Drozdowicz D, Kwiecień S. Are probiotics effective in the treatment of fungal colonization of the gastrointestinal tract? Experimental and clinical studies. *J Physiol Pharmacol.* 2006 Nov;57 Suppl 9:35-49.

Index

abdominal pain, 46
absorption, 45, 57, 86, 89, 90, 96, 105
Acetobacter aceti, 111
Acetobacter xylinoides, 111
Acetobacter xylinum, 111
acid-blockers, 23
acidolin, 26, 89
acidophilus, 110
aciophilin, 26
acquired immunity, 76, 77
Actinomyces sp., 72, 80
actinomycin, 80
adhesion, 59, 92, 95
agave, 105
AIDS, 8, 44, 86, 93
allergies, 1, 11, 40, 43, 52, 54, 56, 57, 58, 75, 91
American Type Culture Collection (ATTC), 98
anorexia nervosa, 68, 69
antacids, 23
antibodies, 23, 24, 76, 90
antigen, 21, 54
anxiety, 68
appendix, 40, 102, 103
arthritis, 4, 11, 58
asparagus, 105
Aspergillus oryzae, 111
asthma, 11, 58, 92
atherosclerosis, 95
atopic dermatitis, 26, 53, 55, 59, 86, 93
autoimmunity, 18, 38, 75
Bacillus cereus, 36
bacterial translocation, 57
bacterlocin, 26
bacteroides, 55, 65
Bacteroides fragilis, 5, 55
B-cells, 21, 23, 24, 25, 29, 31, 32, 41, 43, 118

Belgian endive, 105
beta-glucosidase, 44, 93, 107, 108
beta-glucuronidase, 106, 108
bifidobacteria, 39
Bifidobacterium animalis, 53
Bifidobacterium bifidum, 26, 35, 36, 51, 63, 70
Bifidobacterium infantis, 39, 76
Bifidobacterium lactis, 48, 51, 54, 59, 67, 68, 70, 71, 77
Bifidobacterium longum, 53, 55, 58, 61, 62, 63, 70, 76
bile acids, 43
biotin, 26, 45
Blastocystis hominis, 57
bloating, 44, 45
Borna virus, 6
Borrelia burgdorferi, 3, 5, 82
breast-feeding, 39, 85, 88
bronchitis, 91
Brucella melitensis, 5
Brucellae spp., 5
brush barrier, 57, 58
bulgarican, 26, 36, 95
burn, 51, 94
butter, 14, 111
buttermilk, 111
calcium, 18, 43, 47, 90, 91, 105
Calcivirus, 15
campylobacter, 104
Campylobacter jejuni, 5, 10, 15, 17, 104
cancer, 43, 44, 45, 46, 92, 106, 107, 108
Candida albicans, 4, 11, 26, 43, 58, 60, 64, 66, 87, 89, 90, 92, 97

carcinomatous peritonitis, 92
cardiovascular disease, 4, 11
CD (cluster of differentiation), 44
cell-mediated immune response, 24
cheese, 50, 85, 90, 91, 96, 111
chewable tablets, 99
chickenpox, 9
chicory, 105
Chlamydia pneumoniae, 6, 9
Chlamydia trachomatis, 5
cholera, 18
cholesterol, 45, 86, 89, 90, 92, 94, 95
chronic fatigue syndrome, 4, 11
cilia, 23
clostridia, 5, 11
Clostridium botulinum, 35
Clostridium difficile, 5, 11, 81, 86, 92, 93, 94
Clostridium perfringens, 35, 81
Clostridium tetani, 81
Clostrium botulinum, 17
cobalamine, 45
colic, 67, 86, 88, 93
colitis, 61, 90
Collection Nationale de Cultures de Microorganismes, 98
colon cancer, 92, 93, 106, 107, 108
colony forming units, 99, 100
conjunctiva, 21, 69, 81, 83
constipation, 92, 93
corticosteroids, 117
Corynebacterium diphtheriae, 81

Corynebacterium sp., 81
Corynebacterium striatum, 5
Coxackle B virus, 5
C-reactive protein (CRP), 44, 63, 91
Crohn's disease, 4
Cryptococcal pyarthrosis, 5
cryptosporidiosis, 18
Cryptosporidium, 15
cytokines, 25, 44, 49, 55, 61, 77, 88, 118
Cytomegalovirus, 5
dengue fever, 18
dermatitis, 55, 56
diarrhea, 11, 17, 41, 42, 71, 86, 88, 90, 91, 95
diphtheria, 81
diverticular disease, 91
dyspepsia, 88, 90
ear infection, 10, 67, 93
eczema, 52, 53, 54, 56, 88, 93
electrocardiogram, 28
endotoxins, 38, 42, 46, 52, 58, 69, 106, 116, 119
Enterococcus faecalis, 4, 5, 81
Enterococcus faecium, 13
eosinophilia, 74
epithelium, 27, 57
Escherichia coli, 4, 5, 7, 10, 14, 15, 17, 18, 35, 47, 51, 55, 60, 81, 87, 89, 105
esophagus, 23, 27
essential fatty acids, 44
fatigue, 73
fever, 17, 70, 71, 110
fiber, 44, 58, 117
flatulence, 88, 95
flavonoids, 105
flossing, 113

Mycoplasma pneumoniae, 82
mycoplasmas, 18
nanobacteria, 18
nausea, 17, 44, 88, 95
necrotizing fasciitis, 4, 50
Neisseria gonorrhoeae, 5
Neisseria meningitides, 82
neutrophils, 76
niacin, 26, 45
nitrate, 49
Norwalk-like virus, 15
NSAIDs, 58
nucleic acids, 104
nutrition, 67, 105, 106
Ochrobactrum anthropi, 5
olfactory, 28
oligosaccharides, 104, 105
oral plaque, 47, 49, 50, 84,
    85, 88, 101, 103, 113,
    114, 116
oxygen, 17, 67, 87, 88, 92
pancreatitis, 59
pantothenic acid, 26, 45
papilloma virus (HPV), 5
papillomavirus, 9
parasites, 3
parathyroid hormone, 91
Pasteurella multocida, 5
pasteurization, 16, 17, 18,
    19, 110
pathobiotic, 39
p-cresol, 107
Pediococcus pentosaceus, 74
peptidoglycans, 26, 43
Peptococcaceae, 79
periodontal disease, 42, 47,
    48, 84, 87, 96, 113, 114,
    115
pertussis, 9
pesticides, 58
phagocytic cells, 25

pharmaceuticals, 7, 25, 41,
    57, 58, 89
phenol, 107
phospholipids, 60
phytonutrients, 106
Picha fermentans, 111
picornavirus, 6
pituitary gland, 28
plasmid, 12, 13, 14, 98
Pneumocystis jiroveci, 5
pneumonia, 4, 18, 46, 70,
    73, 74, 75, 91, 95
Pneumonococcal aerogenes,
    4, 5
polarity, 27
polio, 9
polyphenols, 105
polyps, 44
Porphyromonas gingivalis, 3,
    4, 5, 47, 72
prebiotics, 54, 71, 74, 104,
    105, 109
Prevotella bivia, 5
Prevotella intermedia, 4, 5,
    47
Prevotella loescheii, 5
Prevotella sp., 72
probiotic supplementation,
    52, 53, 54, 55, 56, 59, 64,
    73, 75, 76, 77, 97, 98, 99,
    100, 107, 108, 115, 116,
    117, 119
*Propionibacterium
    freudenreichii*, 26, 54
prostaglandins, 45
Proteus mirabilis, 35
Proteus sp., 81
Pseudomonas, 26, 97
Pseudomonas aeruginosa, 5,
    74, 82, 91, 93

Printed in Great Britain
by Amazon.co.uk, Ltd.,
Marston Gate.